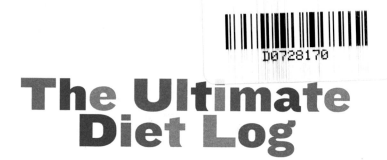

The Ultimate Diet Log

The Ultimate Diet Log

A Unique Food and Exercise Diary
That Fits Any Weight-loss Plan

SUZANNE SCHLOSBERG

AND

CYNTHIA SASS, MPH, MA, RD, CSSD

HOUGHTON MIFFLIN HARCOURT

Boston New York

2009

For information about permission
to reproduce selections from this book, write to
Permissions, Houghton Mifflin Harcourt Publishing Company,
215 Park Avenue South, New York, New York 10003.

www.hmhbooks.com

Library of Congress Cataloging-in-Publication Data

Schlosberg, Suzanne.
The ultimate diet log : a unique food and exercise diary that fits any weight-loss
plan / Suzanne Schlosberg and Cynthia Sass.
p. cm.
ISBN-13: 978-0-618-96895-4
ISBN-10: 0-618-96895-4
1. Weight loss—Diaries. 2. Logbooks. I. Sass, Cynthia. II. Title.
RM222.2.S277 2009
613.2'5—dc22   2008038791

Book design by Lisa Diercks
Typeset in The Serif.

DOC 10 9 8 7 6 5 4

This book includes information about a variety of topics related to diet, exercise, and health. The ideas and suggestions contained in this book are not intended as a substitute for the services of a trained professional or the advice of a medical expert. The authors and publisher disclaim responsibility for any adverse effects resulting directly or indirectly from information contained in this book.

Contents

that the diners ate nearly 30 percent more bread than they thought they'd eaten. Remarkably, 12 percent of the bread eaters denied having touched any bread at all.

That's because eating, while obviously a conscious act, is often mindless too. When you're ingesting calories, you're usually multitasking. You're wolfing down a sandwich while checking e-mail, you're devouring a pizza while catching up with your kids, or you're inhaling a smoothie while navigating rush-hour traffic on your commute to work. Eating, in fact, is a lot like driving. Just as you don't remember stepping on the brake each time you make a right turn, you don't recall each time you dip into that basket of tortilla chips at a Mexican restaurant.

What's more, we tend to have selective memories. We recall our successful days, when we enjoyed a turkey sandwich on whole-wheat bread for lunch and snacked on low-fat popcorn, and we conveniently forget the days when we scarfed down a burger and fries, then indulged in a maple scone and a 20-ounce blended mocha. Emphasizing the positive is just human nature. But too often, our fuzzy memory blinds us to reality. In a recent telephone survey of 12,000 people, for instance, 73 percent of obese respondents told the interviewers that their diet was either "very healthy" or "somewhat healthy" — clearly not an accurate assessment considering their weight!

In our experience — Cynthia's fifteen years as a practicing dietitian and Suzanne's fifteen years as a health writer — we've found that virtually everyone believes they eat more nutritiously than they actually do. Cynthia's clients frequently make comments like "I eat tons of fruits and vegetables" or "I hardly ever snack," only to learn, via a food diary, that their perceptions were completely off base.

A food and exercise diary is, simply, the most powerful tool we know of for making lasting lifestyle changes. Monitoring your habits is like turning up the lights and peering into one of those magnifying mirrors that facialists use: you really see what's going on, in ways that simply weren't apparent before. "Almost everyone who does it is going to lose weight," says Rob Carels, Ph.D., a psychology professor at Bowling Green State University, who has researched the benefits of maintaining food and exercise diaries. "It can be the difference between being successful and not."

The more diligently you record your habits, Carels has found, the more success you're likely to have. In one study, Carels discovered that the successful losers—those who shed at least 5 percent of their body weight over three months—kept food and exercise diaries on eighty-one days, virtually every day of the study. Those who failed to meet the 5 percent goal tracked their habits on only thirty-five days. In another trial, this one lasting six months, Carels reported that overweight adults who maintained a daily workout diary lost twenty-three pounds and averaged nearly three hours of exercise a week. Those who didn't log their workouts lost twelve pounds and averaged just ninety minutes of weekly exercise.

More evidence: a study from Kaiser Permanente's Center for Health Research found that keeping a food diary can double a person's weight loss. In that study, published in the *American Journal of Preventive Medicine,* participants who kept daily food records lost eighteen pounds over six months, compared to nine pounds for those who kept no records. One of the study's authors called keeping a food diary "hands down, the most successful weight-loss method."

Food and exercise diaries work because they keep you honest. Suddenly, you can't fool yourself about how much saturated fat or how few whole grains you eat. What's more, your log will reveal patterns in your habits—clues that might explain why you're not dropping pounds at the rate you expected. You might discover, for example, that you tend to skip breakfast on Fridays or walk 25 percent fewer steps on weekends. Armed with this knowledge, you can take measures to improve your habits.

When you actually see on paper that you're eating sweets twice a day rather than a few times a week, as you assumed, the awareness to stay on track, the way you might continue to balance your checkbook even though you're out of debt with plenty of savings in your account.

Good luck! We welcome your feedback.

Suzanne Schlosberg
suzanne@suzanneschlosberg.com

Cynthia Sass, MPH, MA, RD, CSSD
cynthia@cynthiasass.com

Six-Month Goals and Results

The goals page on the inside cover of this book is the place to consider the big picture: where you stand now and what you'd like to accomplish over the next six months.

When you're trying to make significant lifestyle changes, you need a mental map, but the scope has to be perfect. Imagining where you want to end up a year from now can be overwhelming, and possibly so removed from your starting point that it's too hard to visualize or relate to. On the flip side, concentrating only on the very next step, like what you'll accomplish today or this week, can keep you moving at a snail's pace, because your focus is too narrow to challenge you. Establishing both short-term and six-month goals is like a Goldilocks approach: it's just right. Half a year is close enough to feel attainable, yet distant enough for you to realize you have to get serious in order to get there on time. Once you set your six-month goals, zeroing in on the nitty-gritty tasks you'll track daily will keep you focused, bringing your plan to life.

At the end of twenty-six weeks, return to the goals page and see how your goals matched up with your results. If you stick with this diary, you'll be amazed at how far you've come. Following are tips for filling out each section of the page.

whose certification includes blood-pressure training. However, even supermarket tests are relatively accurate and can let you know if you're in the healthy range. Weight loss, exercise, stress reduction, and limiting sodium and saturated fat in your diet all can help lower your blood pressure, as can prescription medications.

MEASUREMENTS

Watching your body measurements shrink can be highly motivating. For determining health risk, the most important measurement is your waist. Women with a waist larger than 35 inches are at greater risk for obesity-related diseases, according to the National Institutes of Health. For men, the critical number is 40 inches.

FITNESS ASSESSMENTS

Use this section to track any number of fitness tests, such as how fast you can walk one mile, how many pushups you can do, how much weight you can bench press, how far you can stretch your hamstrings, and so on. If you sign up with a fitness trainer, you'll undergo a whole battery of assessments.

EXERCISE HABITS

Here you can summarize your habits, such as how many steps you typically take in a day (wear a pedometer for three straight days and take an average), how often you walk or work out at the gym each week, and so on. Studies show that most of us overestimate how much exercise we do, so be honest!

EATING HABITS

For "areas that need improvement," look at the results of your five-day personal inventory on page 21.

Filling Out
Your Daily Log

Remember, this is *your* log! You can make as many, or as few, notes as you want. Although the format offers plenty of structure, you needn't fill in every box every day. The amount of information you track probably will vary over time. You may go through periods when you want to record your diet and exercise program in minute detail, from the time of day you ate each meal to your emotions at each meal to the number of steps you walked each day. At other times, you may simply want to track your fruit intake. Just make sure you track *something* every day so that you maintain the habit of self-monitoring. The more frequently you record your habits, research shows, the more likely you are to succeed in changing them.

Before starting your daily log, we recommend that you complete the exercise titled "Analyzing Your Diet: A Five-Day Personal Inventory," which starts on page 21. This undertaking will help you decide which dietary habits to focus on, whether it's your intake of trans fat, sodium, fiber, fruit, or sweetened beverages. However, if you're already certain about where you want to concentrate your efforts, skip the evaluation and dive right into the daily log.

Following are tips for filling out each section of your log. Experiment with the format, and eventually you'll find the system that works best for you.

GOALS FOR THE WEEK

At the beginning of each week, set two nutrition goals related to your focus areas and one exercise goal. These goals should be specific and measurable. For example, rather than aim to "cut back on sweets," set a goal to "limit to one sweet per day" or "switch from Frappuccinos to nonfat mochas." Instead of "exercise more," write "walk for 40 min./3 days" or "take 2 Pilates classes."

Make sure your goals are sensible! If you discovered in the five-day assessment that you average just 12 grams of fiber per day, don't suddenly shoot for 30; at this point, 20 would be a more practical goal. If you typically exercise twice a week, aim for three sessions rather than six.

You needn't push yourself to new heights every week. Sometimes, it's best to stick with the same goal for several weeks, or even months, until the practice becomes a habit and you're ready to reach for the next level. At other times, however, you might be in the mood to really test yourself. Maybe this is the week you're determined to average four vegetable servings per day! Also consider your personality. Some people succeed when their goals are moderately challenging whereas others thrive when they shoot for the stars.

GOALS FOR THE WEEK

Let's say your focus areas are skipping meals and whole grains. Your goals for the week could be:

> Eat breakfast 5 days, average 3 whole grains/day, walk 30 min. on treadmill/4 days at level 3.5.

Or

> Bring lunch to work every day, eat whole-grain waffles or cereal for breakfast, try a Spinning class this weekend.

If your focus areas are saturated fat and vegetables, your goals for the week could be:

Switch from 2% to skim milk, eat carrots w/lunch and salad w/dinner M-F, do 2 yoga videos.

Or

Switch to 99% lean ground beef, switch from blue cheese to balsamic vinaigrette dressing, buy light microwave popcorn instead of chips, walk 15 min. during lunch break M-F.

SUPPLEMENTS/MEDICATIONS

If you take a daily multivitamin, calcium supplement, or doctor-prescribed medication, use these boxes to record your supplements or meds. Otherwise, leave the boxes blank.

Note that if you follow the Food Guide Pyramid every day, you don't need a multivitamin or any single vitamin or mineral supplement. But since you bought this book, you're probably at least a few steps away from consistently fitting in every recommended serving of whole grains, veggies, fruits, low-fat dairy, and so on. So you may have a nutrient gap, in which case a multivitamin or mineral supplement may help patch up your nutrient intake. If you choose to take a multi, look for one with no more than 100 percent of the Daily Value for any vitamin or mineral, and skip the extras like green tea and added antioxidants or phytochemicals. Some studies have shown a health risk related to taking isolated antioxidants in pill form, and there's no research to support their benefit.

Finally, keep in mind that a daily supplement is no panacea for inadequate eating habits. A panel of nutrition experts commissioned by the National Institutes of Health concluded that people who pop a daily pill don't have a reduced disease risk.

WEIGHT

Do you really need to weigh yourself daily? No, but use this box if you want to.

How often you should weigh yourself is a matter of some controversy and may depend on your personality. Some experts believe that it's best to step on the scale at most once a week or even once a month, since daily weigh-ins can reinforce an obsession with weight. Frequent weigh-ins also can be misleading because weight can fluctuate from day to day and may not reflect actual fat loss or gains. For example, just two cups of water weigh one pound, so if you're retaining fluid, your weight can jump by several pounds within a twenty-four-hour period, even if your actual fat and muscle mass have remained steady.

On the other hand, some research suggests that people who weigh themselves daily are better able to control their weight than those who step on the scale less frequently. Daily weigh-ins may help you nip a problem in the bud. If you wait a month to weigh yourself, you might discover that, oops, you've gained several pounds and will have a bigger job ahead of you.

If you do weigh yourself daily—a practice we endorse!—do it at the same time each day, and don't get discouraged if the number increases on any particular day. It's more important to look at the big picture. (You can track your weekly weight loss using the chart on page 285.) If you notice your weight creeping up over a two-week period, take action ASAP, before the pounds really pile on. Glance back through your log and analyze where you got off track. Maybe that daily mocha with whipped cream snuck back into your life, or perhaps you made too many trips to the office vending machine.

Also, keep in mind that if your exercise program involves lifting fairly heavy weights, you may be gaining muscle while losing fat, and the scale may not reflect your true progress. Pay attention to whether your clothes are getting looser, and consider getting your body fat tested every few months.

TODAY'S GOALS

Jot down a goal or two first thing in the morning. Make sure your goals are concrete so that at the end of the day, in the Daily Wrap-Up section, you can note definitively whether you met your goals. Here are some sample daily goals:

snack on apple and peanut butter instead of scone
add veggies to my omelet
take stairs at work instead of elevator
eat yogurt & berries instead of ice cream for dessert

MEAL TIME

In the Meal column, indicate what time you ate each meal or snack. This information is most helpful for people who tend to go too long—say, more than five hours—without eating. If you regularly let yourself become ravenous, you are likely to overeat at your next meal and may lose control for the rest of the day.

Tracking meal times can help you determine the best eating pattern to keep you feeling satisfied. For example, maybe you eat dinner at 6 P.M., go to sleep at 11 P.M., and refrain from eating an after-dinner snack, then wake up in the middle of the night hungry. Perhaps eating fruit and/or yogurt at 10 P.M. will enable you to sleep soundly. (It's a myth that anything you eat after 7 P.M. turns to fat!) What matters is how many calories you consume over a twenty-four-hour period, not *when* you eat them. Experiment and find a meal pattern that works for you.

HUNGER/FULLNESS

There are various ways to fill in this section. You can use the rating system described in "Analyzing Your Diet: A Five-Day Personal Inventory," on page 21. This system goes from an *R* (ravenous) to an *S* (stuffed). Or, you can come up with a numerical system that feels right to you, such as −5 (starving) to 5 (your pants are going to burst). Or, to really reinforce this point, you can describe how hungry or full you are in words and phrases, such as "so hungry I'm lightheaded," "perfectly satisfied," or "a little too full."

Whatever method you choose, this is important information to jot

In addition, for cardio activities such as walking, swimming, or using the elliptical trainer, note the distance you covered, your pace (say, 4.2 mph on the treadmill), and your workout intensity (how hard you pushed). You can indicate your intensity with words ("took it easy" or "killer workout!") or a scale from 1 to 10, 1 being so easy that you could easily belt out show tunes while you exercise and 10 being so hard that you're about to keel over. Aim for a mix of longer, slower workouts and shorter, tougher sessions. Most of your workouts should be in the 5 to 8 range.

Consider recording additional aspects of your workout, such as how you felt, your workout partners, and the weather. Perhaps you enjoy exercise more when you take yoga with a certain instructor or hike with a particular friend. If you're using a pedometer to track your activity level, this is the place to indicate your step count for the day.

When recording strength-training workouts, you could write "total-body circuit" or "body-sculpting class," or you could jot down each exercise you did.

EXERCISE

lunchtime walk w/Brenda
35 min., brisk pace
total steps today: 9,683

Or

Bike, 20 min., L 6 hills—pushed hard!
Abs: crunches w/ball—3 sets each

DAILY WRAP-UP

This box holds you accountable for the goals you set each day. Simply check off whether you exceeded your goals, met them, or need to "keep trying." There's also space for a brief note about the day.

Goals: Met ___ **Exceeded** _X_ **Keep Trying** ___

best fiber day yet—25g!
awesome kickboxing class

SUCCESS OF THE DAY
Even if your day was a dietary disaster—you gobbled down a whole pint of Ben & Jerry's Cherry Garcia while glued to *American Idol*—give yourself credit for doing something right, whether it was walking for twenty minutes before breakfast or ordering nonfat milk instead of whole milk in your latte.

WEEKLY WRAP-UP
Here's your chance to look back at the week you just completed. Recording how much you accomplished one week can get you psyched as you start the next.

GOALS ASSESSMENT
This section nudges you to look back at the goals you set the previous Monday. If you consistently fall short, perhaps you have unrealistic expectations; make a note about why you think you didn't meet your goals. On the other hand, if you frequently exceed your goals, maybe you need more of a challenge. If you're usually right on target, congratulations! You have a good sense of the type of goals that work for you.

EXERCISE NOTES
Assess your week as a whole, indicating how many days you exercised, the total number of hours/minutes you spent working out, and any other relevant information, such as your average step count.

PROGRESS REPORT
Use this section to reflect on the past week, answering these questions:

The more accurate your records, the more useful the results will be. Keep your log with you at all times over these five days so that you record your intake as it happens and not from memory.

STEP I: FILLING OUT YOUR FIVE-DAY PERSONAL INVENTORY

Following are instructions for filling in each section of the chart.

➡ **Food/Beverage Amount:** Record everything you eat and drink over five days. We mean *everything*—each handful of nuts you munched on at a party, the soda you sucked down at the movies, the three caramel candies you grabbed from the bowl at the mortgage broker's office. Be specific. Write "½ cup Yoplait nonfat vanilla yogurt and 1 large apple" rather than simply "yogurt, apple." You'll need these details for Step Two, which involves converting your food diary into "trackable units," such as grams of saturated fat, milligrams of sodium, servings of whole grains, and so on.

Use the Personal Inventory pages (pages 26–35) to note relevant details from food containers or wrappers. For example, after you eat that bag of potato chips, jot down the calories, saturated, fiber, sodium, and so on listed on the package. With major brands, you also can find this information online, at websites such as www.calorie-count.com, or on the manufacturer's website. However, you might find it easier to make the notes while you have the packaging handy. For food items that don't come with labels—like an apple, a chicken breast, or a Denver omelet—you can find nutrient data on the U.S. Department of Agriculture's nutrient database, www.nal.usda.gov/fnic/foodcomp/search/, in numerous books, and at www.calorie-count.com or www.calorie king.com. You may have to make some educated guesses.

➡ **Eating Environment:** Note where and with whom you ate, as well as what you were doing when you dined. Did you eat breakfast alone while reading the newspaper? Did you scarf down lunch at your desk between phone calls with clients? Did you eat dinner at home with your family while watching *Survivor,* or did you have a leisurely meal with your spouse at a romantic restaurant?

▶ **Emotions:** Record your emotions, before, during, and after each meal or snack. When you drank that large pumpkin spice iced latte at Dunkin' Donuts, were you feeling stressed from a rough day at work? Did you feel calmer with each sip? Afterward did you feel happy? Guilty?

▶ **Hunger Rating:** Before and after each meal, rate your hunger according to the following scale.

R = RAVENOUS. You're shaky and irritable and will probably eat the first thing you see, quickly and in great quantities.

M = MODERATELY HUNGRY. You have some physical symptoms of hunger such as a growling tummy or a low-energy feeling, but you're not ravenous.

F = FULL BUT NOT SATISFIED. Your physical symptoms of hunger are gone, but you don't feel satisfied by what you ate. It just didn't "do it" for you.

J = JUST RIGHT. You feel full but not overly so. You feel satisfied and ready to move on with your day, but you also feel energized, like you could do cartwheels down the sidewalk.

T = TOO FULL. You overdid it and feel like a bump on a log. You have that heavy, lethargic, brick-in-your-stomach feeling.

S = STUFFED. You want to change into elastic-waistband pants, curl up into a ball, and wait for the pressure to subside. You may even need a few antacids. Ugh!

▶ **Post-meal Insights:** As you reflect on your meal experience — what, where, when, and especially *why* you ate — do any light bulbs go off? For example, maybe you overate because a friend or family member encouraged you to have seconds or split a dessert, or maybe your grandmother's "clean your plate" mandate still rings in your ears. Or maybe your lack of planning led you to eat junk food for dinner.

SAMPLE PERSONAL INVENTORY

	Food/Drink and Amount	Eating Environment
BREAKFAST 7 (a.m.)/p.m.	Coke, 1 20 oz bottle	In car alone
SNACK 10:20 (a.m.)/p.m.	Half an onion bagel with 2 Tbsp veggie cream cheese, 6 oz OJ	Break room at the office, chatting with coworkers
LUNCH 1:45 a.m./(p.m.)	Frozen Amy's black bean vegetable enchiladas microwave dinner, pineapple fruit cup, 16 oz bottled water	At desk, alone
SNACK 5:30 a.m./(p.m.)	2 big spoonfuls of peanut butter off spoon	At desk, alone, from pb stash in desk drawer
DINNER 8:40 a.m./(p.m.)	About 1 cup of pasta w/ 1/2 cup jarred sauce, about 2 Tbsp Parmesan cheese, 6 frozen turkey meatballs	In front of TV, alone, with cat
SNACK 11:30 a.m./(p.m.)	Handful of chocolate graham crackers, 4 oz skim milk	Standing in kitchen, alone

Emotions	Hunger Rating	Post-Meal Insights
Frenzied, running late, didn't want to go to work!	Before: F, still full from last night	Shouldn't have had the extra pizza last night. Wasn't hungry for breakfast but I needed "cola buzz"
Stressed! Not enough time in the day	Before: M After: J	A little hungry but mostly just needed a break; felt guilty eating bagel and cream cheese b/c not the healthiest choice but at least only ate half
Not as stressed as a.m. because started to get caught up	Before: M After: J	Felt good about this meal; enjoyed it and wasn't stuffed after
Cranky. Needed a pb fix	Before: R After: M	I could have had one spoonful but it was so good and I needed treat. Just realized I haven't had anything to drink since lunch
Relaxed	Before: M After: T	Ate too much but couldn't stop—it was so warm and hearty
Tired but craving something sweet	Before: F After: T	Wasn't hungry, I just wanted something sweet. The graham crackers weren't even good, prob. b/c looking for a mental treat after a tough day

FIVE-DAY PERSONAL INVENTORY, DAY I

	Food/Drink and Amount	Eating Environment
BREAKFAST _____ a.m./p.m.		
SNACK _____ a.m./p.m.		
LUNCH _____ a.m./p.m.		
SNACK _____ a.m./p.m.		
DINNER _____ a.m./p.m.		
SNACK _____ a.m./p.m.		

Emotions	Hunger Rating	Post-Meal Insights

FIVE-DAY PERSONAL INVENTORY, DAY 3

	Food/Drink and Amount	Eating Environment
BREAKFAST _____ a.m./p.m.		
SNACK _____ a.m./p.m.		
LUNCH _____ a.m./p.m.		
SNACK _____ a.m./p.m.		
DINNER _____ a.m./p.m.		
SNACK _____ a.m./p.m.		

Emotions	Hunger Rating	Post-Meal Insights

FIVE-DAY PERSONAL INVENTORY, DAY 5

	Food/Drink and Amount	Eating Environment
BREAKFAST ____ a.m./p.m.		
SNACK ____ a.m./p.m.		
LUNCH ____ a.m./p.m.		
SNACK ____ a.m./p.m.		
DINNER ____ a.m./p.m.		
SNACK ____ a.m./p.m.		

Emotions	Hunger Rating	Post-Meal Insights

WHOLE GRAINS

Trackable unit =

1 cup dry whole-grain cold cereal such as Cheerios or Kashi (think tennis ball)

½ cup cooked grains like hot oatmeal, wild rice, and whole-wheat pasta (think half a tennis ball)

1 standard slice of whole-grain bread or a bread product (think half a whole-grain English muffin or bun)

Ideal = At least 3

Day	Check number of trackable units each day	Daily total	+ or − above or below ideal
1			
2			
3			
4			
5			

LEAN PROTEIN

Skinless white-meat chicken, grilled fish, beef or pork sirloin, tofu, beans or edamame, or meat substitutes such as a veggie burger.

Trackable unit =

3 oz. cooked (think deck of cards in thickness and width)

½ cup beans (think half a tennis ball)

Ideal = At least 2

Day	Check number of trackable units each day	Daily total	+ or − above or below ideal
1			
2			
3			
4			
5			

PLANT-BASED FATS

Trackable unit =

1 tsp. oil (think 1 die)

1 Tbsp. oil-based salad dressing (think tip of your thumb)

2 Tbsp. light oil-based dressing, nuts, seeds, peanut or almond
butter, chopped avocado (think 2 thumb tips)

Ideal = About 3

Day	Check number of trackable units each day	Daily total	+ or – above or below ideal
1			
2			
3			
4			
5			

FIBER

Trackable unit = Gram of fiber

Ideal = 25 grams per day for women, 36 grams per day for men

Day	Record # of grams you ate each day	Daily total	+ or – above or below ideal
1			
2			
3			
4			
5			

LOW-FAT DAIRY/CALCIUM SOURCE

Low-fat or nonfat yogurt; 1 percent, skim, or calcium-fortified soy milk; reduced-fat string, brick, shredded, sliced, or crumbled cheese; cottage or ricotta cheese.

Trackable unit =

1 cup or 8 oz. milk or yogurt (think 1-cup measuring cup)

1 piece string cheese

1 slice cheese (think coaster)

¼ cup shredded or crumbled cheese (think golf ball)

1 oz. brick cheese (think 4 dice)

½ cup cottage or ricotta cheese (think half a tennis ball)

Ideal = About 3

Day	Check number of trackable units each day	Daily total	+ or – above or below ideal
1			
2			
3			
4			
5			

NOT-SO-HEALTHY-STUFF TALLY

In this section tally your intake of the food categories that most of us need to limit: sweetened beverages, refined grains, saturated and trans fats, sweets, sodium, alcohol, and calories. You'll also track the detrimental habits that many of us need to reform: overeating, skipping meals, and emotional eating.

SWEETENED BEVERAGES

Soda, lemonade, fruit punch, sweetened tea, caffé mocha.

Trackable unit =

1 cup or 8 oz. (think 1-cup measuring cup)

Ideal = 0

Day	Check number of trackable units each day	Daily total	+ or – above or below ideal
1			
2			
3			
4			
5			

REFINED GRAINS

Trackable unit =

1 cup dry sugary cold cereal (think tennis ball)

½ cup cooked grains like white rice and white pasta (think half a tennis ball)

1 standard-size slice of white bread or bread product (think half an English muffin or bun)

Ideal = 0

Day	Check number of trackable units each day	Daily total	+ or - above or below ideal
1			
2			
3			
4			
5			

SATURATED AND TRANS FAT

Trackable unit = Gram of saturated or trans fat

Ideal = Fewer than 22 grams per day (saturated and trans fat combined)

Day	Record number of grams each day	Daily total	+ or - above or below ideal
1			
2			
3			
4			
5			

Chocolate candy, sugar candy, cookies, pastries, ice cream.

Trackable unit =

Small handful of candy or one cookie the size of your palm or two cookies the size of the bottom of a soda can

½ cup ice cream (think half a tennis ball)

1 cup frozen yogurt (think tennis ball or 1-cup measuring cup)

Ideal = 1

Day	Check number of trackable units each day	Daily total	+ or – above or below ideal
1			
2			
3			
4			
5			

Trackable unit =

Mg of sodium from food labels

count 1 tsp. of table salt (think 1 die) as 2,300 mg; a dash or two quick shakes is about 145 mg of sodium (¹⁄₁₆ of a tsp.)

Ideal = No more than 2,300 mg per day

Day	Record number of mg you had each day	Daily total	+ or – above or below ideal
1			
2			
3			
4			
5			

Trackable unit = Any meal or snack where emotions (stress, boredom, sadness, happiness) rather than hunger affected your choices

Ideal = 0

Day	Check number of meals and snacks driven by emotional eating	Total emotional eating instances	+ or – above or below ideal
1			
2			
3			
4			
5			

STEP 3: ANALYZING YOUR RESULTS

Congratulations! You're almost done with your inventory. Here's where things really get cooking. When you step outside of yourself to objectively fill out an assessment like this one, you get a much closer picture of your daily habits.

Based on your tallies, which are your strongest areas? Where do you consistently exceed the ideal?

1. _____

2. _____

3. _____

In which three Healthy Stuff categories do you need to improve most? In other words, where do you have the most minus marks?

1. _____

2. _____

3. _____

In which three Not-So-Healthy Stuff categories do you need to improve most? In other words, which categories have the most plus marks?

1. _____

2. _____

3. _____

Of the six areas in which you most need to improve, choose four that meet the following criteria:

When you start using your daily log, focus on two areas at a time. Once you see progress or have incorporated the new habits into your life, introduce one or two new focus areas. You may want to switch one or both of your focus areas every few weeks or every few months, depending on your progress. Some habits are easier to reform than others. For example, maybe you can't imagine enjoying a salad unless it's loaded with cheese and creamy dressing—because that's how your mom made it—but switching from 2 percent to nonfat milk in your latte and smoothies might not require much of a sacrifice.

Now that you know which four changes you want to make, it's time to get real. It may or may not be practical for you to make the ideal your goal. For example, if you're currently drinking six trackable units of sweetened beverages a day, can you really go cold turkey? Maybe—or maybe not. The good news is, at least you know where you're starting, and you know the ideal (zero). If you select two or even four as your goal, you're heading in the right direction! Two months from now, you could reset your goal for one sweetened beverage a day.

If you set your sights on a radical overhaul, you may struggle (that's normal). We want you to be successful and feel proud of the changes you're making. So ask yourself (and be really, really honest here): "How much of a change can I realistically make on a daily basis without feeling frustrated, deprived, or overwhelmed?" Keep in mind that you can always modify your goal if it starts to seem exceedingly easy or impossible to achieve.

OK, now that you've thought it through, record your goals below. Then transfer the information to the "Six-Month Goals and Results" page on the inside cover of the book.

GOAL #1

My first focus area is: _____.

I want to go from _____ (trackable units or amount)
to _____.

GOAL #2

My second focus area is: _____.

I want to go from _____ (trackable units or amount)
to _____.

GOAL #3

My third focus area is: _____.

I want to go from _____ (trackable units or amount)
to _____.

GOAL #4

My fourth focus area is: _____.

I want to go from _____ (trackable units or amount)
to _____.

feeling of fullness that whole fruits do. Most of your fruit servings should be whole fruits.

HEALTH BENEFITS
Fruits are rich in fiber, vitamins, minerals, antioxidants, and phytochemicals, helping fight heart disease, cancer, type 2 diabetes, and other diseases. Research shows that eating a variety of produce provides even better protection against disease by reducing oxidation, a chemical process that causes damage and deterioration in the body. (Think of a freshly sliced apple turning brown; that's an example of oxidation, and scientists believe this reaction initiates disease). So branch out from your usual apples, bananas, and oranges and mix in some apricots, dates, kiwis, and persimmons.

WEIGHT-CONTROL BENEFITS
Fruits are filled with water and fiber and therefore promote fullness, helping you cut calories without even trying. Oranges, for instance, are 88 percent water, and apples and pineapples are 85 percent water! (Watermelon, not surprisingly, is 95 percent water.) Research suggests that people who eat the most fruit have lower BMIs that those who eat little fruit.

PRACTICAL TIPS
➡ Add sliced banana or berries to your breakfast cereal or oatmeal. Stirring microwaved frozen berries into oatmeal is a great off-season way to maintain your fruit intake.

➡ Toss fruit into your salad. In a spinach or dark green salad, try strawberries, blueberries, blood oranges, pink grapefruit, cherries, or figs. In field greens or romaine, go with pineapple, mango, apples, pears, plums, or pomegranates.

➡ Make a fruit smoothie for breakfast or a snack. Blend a small fresh or frozen sliced banana and/or 1 cup of frozen berries with 1 cup of skim or soy milk. Keep sliced frozen bananas in the freezer.

⮕ Substitute a baked apple or baked pear for a sugary dessert. Instead of indulging in 1 cup of ice cream for dessert, eat a ½ cup topped with 1 cup of berries, cherries, or sliced peaches.

FOCUS AREA: VEGETABLES

Mom would not be proud: according to the CDC, only 22 percent of men and 32 percent of women eat the recommended three or more vegetable servings per day. If you're not sure how to select or cook a particular veggie, ask the supermarket produce manager or farmer at a farmers' market. A farmers' market is the best place to find in-season vegetables rich in flavor and nutrients, and you know exactly where those squash, peppers, and tomatoes came from. For a list of farmer's markets in your area, check www.ams.usda.gov/farmersmarkets/map .htm.

Frozen veggies also are an excellent option. They're typically frozen within hours of being picked, which means they're allowed to mature before they're harvested, when they're at their peak nutritional value. They may be even more nutritious than fresh vegetables that have spent a week crossing the country on a truck. Be sure that the frozen vegetable package indicates that the only ingredient is the veggie itself and not butter, salt, hydrogenated oils, and artificial colors and preservatives.

HEALTH BENEFITS

Eating your veggies is one of the most important steps you can take to improve your health. Compared to vegetable avoiders, veggie eaters have lower rates of heart disease, type 2 diabetes, certain cancers, kidney stones, bone loss, and obesity. Veggies are chock full of fiber, vitamins, minerals, antioxidants, and phytochemicals.

WEIGHT-CONTROL BENEFITS

Vegetables are both filling and low in calories, which means they can help you cut calories without decreasing your portion sizes. In one

PRACTICAL TIPS

➡ Snack on popcorn instead of pretzels or crackers.

➡ Mix whole oats with peanut butter and raisins, and fill celery sticks with the mixture.

➡ Mix whole oats, chopped nuts, and dried cherries into melted dark chocolate; roll into balls, set on wax paper, and enjoy as a treat.

➡ Mix whole-grain cereal into yogurt as a snack or at breakfast.

➡ Sprinkle toasted oats onto fruit salad or into garden salads.

➡ Add brown or wild rice or whole oats into ground beef or turkey when making burger patties, meatballs, or meatloaf.

➡ Serve whole grains as a side dish by making a chilled grain and veggie salad; combine cooled whole-wheat pasta spirals or wild rice with chopped veggies and light balsamic vinaigrette.

FOCUS AREA: LEAN PROTEIN

Protein is one of the building blocks of every cell in our bodies. We actually lose a certain amount of protein each day as some cells die off. Dietary protein helps us replace those cells and repair the cells and tissues that become damaged through exercise, illness, or injury. Unfortunately, animal protein is also naturally bundled with saturated fat and cholesterol. Very few people eat too little protein. For most of us, the issue is eating too much fatty protein, like ground beef and chicken with the skin.

HEALTH BENEFITS

You'll lower your saturated-fat intake—and therefore reduce your heart-disease risk—if you switch to leaner protein sources such as skinless white-meat chicken, grilled fish, beef or pork sirloin, tofu, beans or edamame, or meat substitutes like a veggie burger. There's also substantial evidence linking a high red-meat intake to colon cancer. People who eat the most red meat—about 5 ounces a day—have a 30 to 40 percent greater colon cancer risk than those who eat about 1 ounce or less a day. Processed lunchmeats, hot dogs, and sausages seem to be the worst offenders.

Plant-based proteins are an excellent option. The government's latest dietary guidelines recommend eating three cups of beans per week. Kidney beans, pinto beans, lima beans, black-eyed peas, and lentils are great protein sources, containing about 15 grams per cup, and provide several key nutrients including iron, zinc, fiber (which animal protein lacks), and folate.

WEIGHT-CONTROL BENEFITS

If you switch from fatty to lean protein sources, you'll save a ton of calories. Consider: a 3.5-ounce serving of 80 percent lean ground beef (a little larger than a deck of cards) contains 271 calories, compared to just 171 calories for a serving of 95 percent lean ground beef; both contain 26 grams of protein. A 3-ounce serving of tilapia also contains 26 grams of protein but only 128 calories.

Will eating more protein help you lose weight? That's debatable. In many studies, subjects on high-protein diets do shed more pounds than people on low-fat diets, but the weight loss is typically short-lived and not substantial. For some people, boosting protein intake can help with weight loss by increasing satisfaction. For example, if you usually have a bagel and orange juice for breakfast, you'll probably find yourself satisfied longer by oatmeal made with skim or soy milk topped with almonds, or a breakfast sandwich made with scrambled egg whites, low-fat cheese, and veggies on a whole-wheat English muffin.

PRACTICAL TIPS

➡ Add three or four slices of lean deli meat or veggie deli slices to grilled cheese, or roll up and eat the slices as a side dish.

➡ Replace 80 to 85 percent lean ground meats with 99 percent lean ground meats, diced or shredded grilled chicken breast, or tuna canned in water.

➡ Sauté with oil instead of butter.

➡ When baking, replace butter or margarine with a combination of oil and mashed fruit, such as mashed banana, or dried plum, date, or fig purée. For each tablespoon of butter, use 1 teaspoon oil and 2 teaspoons fruit purée.

➡ Use oil-based dressings and vinaigrettes instead of creamy dressings, or dress salads in balsamic or red wine vinegar and sprinkle with chopped nuts or seeds.

➡ Use avocado or guacamole instead of sour cream or cream cheese in wraps or Mexican food.

FOCUS AREA: LOW-FAT DAIRY/CALCIUM-RICH FOODS

The dietary guidelines recommend three daily servings of low-fat dairy to get the broad range of nutrients this food group provides, including protein, calcium, vitamin D, and potassium.

If you can't or don't want to consume dairy products, choose calcium-fortified milk alternatives. We recommend soy or hemp milk, which provide about the same amount of protein and calcium as cow's milk. Other calcium-rich, non-dairy foods include almonds (100 mg per quarter), calcium-fortified juice, cereals, dark greens (collard, spinach, turnip, kale, and bok choy contain 150 to 350 mg per cup), dried figs (135 mg for 5 medium), and fish with soft edible bones (sardines and wild Alaskan salmon contain about 200 mg per 3-ounce portion).

HEALTH BENEFITS

If you're short on dairy and not making a conscious effort to replace it with calcium-fortified products, you may be lacking in calcium, essential for healthy bones, as well as potassium, which helps lower blood pressure.

WEIGHT-CONTROL BENEFITS

You may have heard about a link between dairy intake and weight control. The theory is that calcium somehow prevents fat storage by regulating a hormone or enzyme. We feel that the research is a little shaky, since some studies have found the opposite, linking more dairy to weight gain. But this much is certain: if you switch from whole or 2 percent dairy products to 1 percent or nonfat, you will save big time on calories. One cup of whole milk contains 146 calories, compared to 86 calories for one cup of skim. Also, full-fat and even 2 percent dairy products are too high in saturated fat, the type that increases the risk of heart disease. A single cup of whole milk contains a whopping 5 grams of saturated fat, nearly a quarter of the daily max.

If you're lactose intolerant, purchase fat-free or 1 percent Lactaid milk (real milk without the lactose). If you're mildly lactose intolerant, you can probably consume reduced-fat cheeses and yogurt, since most of the lactose is removed in processing.

PRACTICAL TIPS:

➡ Drink an ice-cold glass of skim, 1 percent, or soy milk as a snack, or blend it with a cup of frozen fruit for a creamy smoothie.

➡ Layer nonfat yogurt or cottage cheese with fresh fruit or fruit canned in 100 percent juice, and sprinkle with chopped nuts for a dessert or snack.

➡ Snack on string cheese or a few cubes of cheese along with a small handful of whole-grain crackers.

➡ Melt cheese onto whole-grain toast and top with fresh sliced tomatoes as a snack.

➡ Spread cottage or ricotta cheese onto whole-grain toast and sprinkle with cinnamon or cloves, or top with berries, sliced peaches or plums, drained canned peaches, mandarin oranges, or pineapple.

FOCUS AREA: FIBER

Fiber is a catchall term for indigestible substances found only in plant foods. There are two types of dietary fiber: soluble and insoluble. Solu-

▣ Serve bean soup as an appetizer or side dish. Canned black bean, lentil, and split pea soups can provide as much as 7 to 10 grams of fiber per cup.

▣ Swap regular pasta for whole wheat. A half cup of cooked whole-wheat pasta typically provides about 6 grams of fiber, compared to 1 to 2 grams in traditional pasta.

FOCUS AREA: SWEETENED BEVERAGES

Sweetened beverages are drinks made with added sugars—in other words, sugars that aren't there naturally. One hundred percent fruit juice isn't considered a sweetened beverage because the sugar is naturally present in the fruit, but fruit punch is a sweetened beverage because most of its sugar is added, in the form of high-fructose corn syrup, the same sweetener used in soda. Other sweetened beverages include lemonade, chocolate milk, coffee drinks made with flavored syrups, and sports or energy drinks.

These days, Americans consume 150 to 300 more calories per day than we did in the 1970s, and 50 percent of that increase has come from sweetened beverages. We now consume 21 percent of our total calories from drinks, about 464 calories per day, and the biggest source is soda. Ideally, we should be getting more like 10 percent—and most of that from low-fat or nonfat milk.

When you scan the nutrition labels of beverages, skip over products that contain the following ingredients: brown sugar, corn sweetener, corn syrup, dextrose, evaporated cane juice, fructose, fruit juice concentrates, glucose, lactose, maltose, sucrose, high-fructose corn syrup, honey, molasses, and raw sugar.

HEALTH BENEFITS

Sweetened beverages are typically just empty calories. If you replace those calories with something more nutritious—say, eating a tangerine instead of sipping sweetened iced tea—you'll be packing more vitamins, minerals, and antioxidants into your diet. Cutting back on or eliminating soda and sweet drinks can reduce the chances of weight gain and, as a result, the incidence of type 2 diabetes.

WEIGHT-CONTROL BENEFITS

Cutting back on sweetened drinks is one of the best ways to lose weight. Research suggests that the brain simply doesn't register liquid calories with our appetite controls. In other words, when you drink a soda, you don't compensate by eating less food.

The next time you're at the market, check out the nutrition facts label on a bottle of soda or sweet tea or lemonade. Compare the calorie and carbohydrate content (which includes sugars) to other foods. For example, one slice of bread provides about 60 calories, from roughly 15 grams of carbohydrate. That's the same amount of carbs in just 5 ounces of soda. The point isn't that carbs are bad but to give you a frame of reference. Your body needs only so much carbohydrate to meet its fuel needs. Soda carbs aren't filling, but solid carbs are. So why "spend" one half to one third of your daily carb allotment on soda?

PRACTICAL TIPS

➡ If you're a sweet tea drinker, wean yourself gradually. Combine sweet tea with unsweetened tea in a 50/50 mixture, then week by week reduce the sweetened portion until it's all unsweetened.

➡ With flavored coffee beverages like mochas or vanilla lattes, gradually decrease the number of syrup pumps added to your drink.

➡ Use money as your motivation! If you purchase one 20-ounce bottle of soda per day, you probably spend about $37.50 per month. Kicking a bottle-a-day habit saves $450 per year.

➡ If the taste of plain water bores you, flavor it with sliced fruit, such as lemon, lime, orange, or pineapple. Or freeze 100 percent juice and bits of real fruit, like raspberries or pineapple, in an ice

PRACTICAL TIPS

To reduce trans fat, eat more fresh foods rather than packaged or fast foods. For example:

➡ Grab a freshly made deli sandwich for lunch instead of a fried chicken sandwich. Fried fast foods are one of the greatest sources of trans fat.

➡ Buy freshly made breads and baked goods instead of packaged.

➡ If you do buy packaged foods, look for those with 0 grams of trans fat and no hydrogenated oils in the ingredient list.

To reduce saturated fat:

➡ Switch from whole milk to skim. It cuts out 5 grams of saturated fat per cup. That's 25 percent of the recommended daily maximum intake.

➡ Switch from 80 percent lean to 95 percent lean ground beef. This cuts out 3 grams of saturated fat per 3 ounces.

➡ Replace one tablespoon of butter with one tablespoon of olive oil. You save 5 grams of saturated fat, another 25 percent of the recommended daily maximum intake.

➡ Watch your portion sizes. A standard portion of shredded cheese is a quarter cup, about the size of a golf ball. Using a quarter cup of shredded cheddar cheese on a salad or burrito instead of a half cup saves you 5 grams of saturated fat, yet another 25 percent of the recommended daily maximum intake.

➡ The next time you eat Mexican, hold the sour cream and ask for guacamole instead. A quarter cup of guacamole made with mashed avocado and seasoning provides only 1 gram of saturated fat, compared to 7 grams in a quarter cup of full-fat sour cream.

➡ Spread peanut butter on toast instead of cream cheese. Of the 8 grams of fat per tablespoon in peanut butter, only 1.5 grams are saturated, compared to 6 of the 9 grams in a tablespoon of cream cheese.

➡ The next time you crave ice cream, head to the ice cream shop for a small soft-serve dish instead of a hard scoop. One half cup of soft-serve vanilla provides only 1.5 grams of saturated fat, compared to 5 grams in a half cup scoop of hard vanilla.

FOCUS AREA: SWEETS

We're talking about chocolate candy, sugar candy, cookies, pastries, other baked goods, and ice cream. We think it's unrealistic and unnecessary to cut these foods out altogether; even the latest dietary guidelines allow for some sweets as part of "discretionary calories," a concept that allows us to "spend" about 200 calories a day on whatever we want, even if it's not so healthy. Of course, you don't have to choose a splurge food every day, but knowing that it's OK can satisfy your cravings so they won't turn into full-on binges.

HEALTH BENEFITS

Aside from being low in fiber and nutrients and high in calories, many sweets are also loaded with trans fat and/or saturated fat, the types that increase cholesterol and the risk of heart disease.

WEIGHT-CONTROL BENEFITS

Sweets are among the highest-calorie foods. A slice of banana walnut loaf at Starbucks contains an astonishing 470 calories. Four macaroons contain 520 calories, and one pint of Häagen-Dazs vanilla chocolate chip ice cream has 1,240 calories!

PRACTICAL TIPS

➡ Instead of keeping ice cream in your fridge, go to a parlor and order one scoop in a cup or a kid's cone. One half cup scoop of Ben & Jerry's Cherry Garcia provides 240 calories, but one pint has 960. The scoop may cost just as much, but it's worth the savings to your waistline and health.

→ Marinate meat in sauces made from fresh juices, such as pineapple with onions and chili peppers, or season with bay leaf, marjoram, sage, mint, and thyme.

→ Add flavor to mashed or baked potatoes with fresh dill, rosemary, or chives and scallions.

→ Season homemade soups or stews and vegetable dishes with fresh or dried basil, bay leaf, dill, marjoram, onion, oregano, parsley, and pepper.

→ Season rice or grain dishes with savory flavors such as cumin, curry powder, onion, and paprika, or spicy seasonings such as ginger, cloves, nutmeg, and cinnamon.

→ Read food labels. Either look at the milligrams of sodium per serving (be sure to multiply this by the number of servings you eat if you eat more than one) or the Percent Daily Value or %DV. The Percent Daily Value is the amount one serving provides compared to the highest amount you should take in per day. One hundred percent of the Daily Value for sodium is set at 2,400 mg, just over the recently revised current recommendation of 2,300 mg per day. If the nutrition facts panel states that one serving of a food provides 25 percent of the Daily Value for sodium, this means one serving provides 25 percent of the 2,400 mg upper limit. The %DV can help you quickly compare similar foods to each other, such as two brands of soup or salad dressing.

FOCUS AREA: ALCOHOL

It's not just alcoholics who should be concerned about their booze intake. If you're trying to lose weight or improve your health, cutting back on alcoholic beverages can make a substantial difference.

HEALTH BENEFITS

Health-wise, alcohol is tricky because it has both pros and cons. In moderation—no more than one drink per day for women or two for men, and no, you can't save them up for the weekend!—drinking alcohol may help reduce the risk of heart disease and stroke. Trouble is, even in moderation, alcohol increases the risk of breast cancer, and above moderation it carries serious health risks, including liver cirrhosis, high blood pressure, liver damage, stroke, damage to the heart and brain, sudden death, accidents, suicide, and cancers of the pancreas, pharynx, larynx, esophagus, and breast. Alcohol affects every cell in the body, and the highest illness and death rates are associated with the highest alcohol intakes.

And, of course, some people shouldn't drink at all, including pregnant and breastfeeding women, children, teens and adults under the legal age limit, people taking medications that interact with alcohol (this includes beta blockers, antidepressants, and blood thinners), and those who have been told to abstain due to their medical status (such as liver or pancreatic disease).

WEIGHT-CONTROL BENEFITS

Alcohol presents a few distinct problems for people who are trying to lose weight. First, alcohol itself contains calories, but the substances it's often mixed with provide even more, especially when those beverages come with little umbrellas. An 8-ounce piña colada contains 437 calories, and some of those frozen, creamy drinks contain upwards of 800 calories!

What's more, even in moderation, alcohol stimulates appetite and lowers inhibitions, which means you're more likely to devour that plate of chicken wings, eat something you probably wouldn't touch sober (cheese fries?), or indulge in a post-celebration, wee-hours-of-the-morning stack of pancakes with butter and syrup.

PRACTICAL TIPS

➡ Order the beverage you'll drink slowest. If you tend to sip wine and guzzle beer, make wine your drink of choice.

➡ Instead of going to happy hour, meet friends at a coffee or tea shop. (But don't order the 600-calorie blended caramel mocha with whipped cream!)

➡ Use lower-calorie condiments that provide rich flavor, such as spicy seeded mustard instead of mayo, balsamic vinegar instead of honey mustard dip, and hummus instead of mayo.

FOCUS AREA: EATING UNTIL OVERLY FULL

When most people think of overeating, the first thing that comes to mind is Thanksgiving, the one day of the year that we seemingly have permission to get really good and stuffed. But many of us overeat to a lesser degree every day, or even multiple times per day.

We stuff ourselves for several reasons, including emotional or stress eating, not wanting to waste food, and even rebound overeating triggered by undereating earlier in the day. To change this pattern, you first have to notice what it feels like to overeat and figure out why you're doing it. Pay close attention to this part of the log and remember: keeping track of what's going on is not about policing yourself or feeling guilty. It's about understanding your patterns so you can change them for good.

HEALTH BENEFITS

Stuffing yourself to the point of discomfort causes bloating, upset stomach, heartburn, sleep troubles, fatigue, and overall sluggishness, all of which can lead to poor work performance or not enjoying social time.

WEIGHT-CONTROL BENEFITS

This one is pretty straightforward: if you stop stuffing yourself, you'll consume fewer calories and shed pounds.

PRACTICAL TIPS

➡ Try eating one meal a day without any distractions such as TV, the Internet, music, or reading material. Just sit at a table and focus on the pace of your eating and the taste and texture of your food. Check in with yourself every five minutes to assess how full you feel.

➡ Eat more slowly. Put down your fork, spoon, or food between each bite, take a deep breath, and relax. This may feel awkward at first, but it's effective in reducing how much you eat.

➡ Ask for a to-go container with your meal. Place half in the container as soon as it arrives on your table, and you've accomplished two things: you'll be less likely to overeat, and you'll save money because now you have two meals for the price of one.

➡ Downsize your plates, bowls, and even utensils. Numerous studies have found that we fill our dishes to whatever size they are, and bigger spoons mean bigger spoonfuls. Use bread plates instead of dinner plates and soup cups instead of bowls.

➡ Don't eat snack foods right out of the bag, box, or jar. Buy single servings or pre-portion them into baggies or sealable containers for the week.

➡ If you find yourself eating for emotional reasons, pause before you eat and identify the emotions that are driving you. Often, this alone has a calming effect. Then try an alternative activity that meets your emotional needs. If you need to talk or vent, call or e-mail a friend. If you need some unconditional love and affection, spend time with a pet. To combat boredom, do a creative project, such as drawing, jewelry making, or playing an instrument.

➡ If your dining companions tend to encourage overeating, ask them to support you by going to restaurants with smaller portions and splitting entrées with you. Or, instead of making plans that revolve around food, invite them to do something active, like going for a hike.

FOCUS AREA: SKIPPING MEALS

People skip meals for all sorts of reasons. For instance, they mistakenly believe that missing a meal will help with weight loss, or they make eating a lower priority than other tasks. Or they're so busy that they simply forget to eat. Our lifestyles nowadays are more hectic than ever. Many of us work more than one job, juggle work and/or volunteer ac-

FOCUS AREA: EMOTIONAL EATING

Many people turn to food when they're bored, tired, overwhelmed, or anxious. Maybe you curl up on the couch with a pint of ice cream when you've had a run-in with a boss or coworker. Or maybe you turn to a blended mocha drink and coffee cake as an energy boost when you're dragging. Or perhaps you try to find pleasure in a pan of brownies when you're unhappy with your job, weight, or relationship. Even happy emotions can trigger eating, like having friends over for dinner when you move into your fabulous new place, or going out to your favorite restaurant after a promotion. To break an emotional-eating pattern, you need to gain awareness of why you're eating, why you've chosen certain foods, and how they're tied to your emotions.

HEALTH BENEFITS

Eating emotionally means taking in calories your body doesn't need, resulting in weight gain, which increases the risk of nearly every chronic disease. And the foods we tend to turn to emotionally are traditionally low in fiber and high in sugar, saturated fat, and sodium. Indulging in ice cream, brownies, or mac and cheese every once in a while is fine, but making it a habit can lead to high blood pressure, high cholesterol, or high blood sugar.

WEIGHT-CONTROL BENEFITS

Overcoming emotional eating can eradicate the number-one source of extra calories in your diet. This one pattern alone may be responsible for several hundred extra calories per day or week, so the payoff for changing it can be substantial.

PRACTICAL TIPS

➡ Before you pick up your fork, zero in on what emotion you're feeling and why. Walk into the other room and really think about it; think of yourself as a detective. Digging down to the root of why you "need" chocolate can help you see that it has nothing to do with food, and that's the first step to changing your pattern. If you're having trouble pinpointing your feelings, Google "list of feelings" so you have a smorgasbord to choose from.

➡ Assess your support system. Do you have enough people in your life to vent to or simply to connect with to talk about your day? Make a conscious effort to strengthen a current relationship or build a new one.

➡ Think about your high-risk situations. When and where are you most prone to eating when you aren't hungry? At home, at work, on the weekends, alone, or with certain people? Think about how you can change your pattern or environment to avoid the emotional-eating land mine. For example, if it tends to happen at night while you watch TV, change your evening routine and join a book club to cut your TV time. Or set up an elliptical trainer in front of your TV.

➡ Build some more "me time" into your day or week. Emotional eating often happens when there is a gap that needs to be filled. Too often the gap is not enough pure fun.

➡ Become compassionate with yourself. Don't call yourself names, like "lazy" or "weak" or "out of control." Instead, remind yourself that you're human and it's impossible to be perfect every minute.

WEEK 1

Goals for the Week: _____

_____

MONDAY

SUPPLEMENTS [ ] [ ]   WEIGHT [ ]

Today's Goals: _____

MEAL	FOODS & BEVERAGES	FOCUS I:	FOCUS 2:
BREAKFAST ___ A.M./P.M.			
Hunger:			
Fullness:			
	MEAL TOTALS		
SNACK ___ A.M./P.M.			
Hunger:			
Fullness:			
	MEAL TOTALS		
LUNCH ___ A.M./P.M.			
Hunger:			
Fullness:			
	MEAL TOTALS		
SNACK ___ A.M./P.M.			
Hunger:			
Fullness:			
	MEAL TOTALS		
DINNER ___ A.M./P.M.			
Hunger:			
Fullness:			
	MEAL TOTALS		
	DAILY TOTALS		

EXERCISE NOTES
_____ minutes

DAILY WRAP-UP
Goals: Exceeded ___ Met ___ Keep Trying ___
Notes:

Success Of The Day:

RESEARCH REPORT: Jumbo food packages prompt you to eat more. In one study, adults given 1-pound M&M bags scarfed down 264 more calories than those given half-pound bags.

TUESDAY

SUPPLEMENTS ☐ ☐   WEIGHT ☐

Today's Goals:

MEAL	FOODS & BEVERAGES	FOCUS I:	FOCUS 2:
BREAKFAST ____ A.M./P.M.			
Hunger:			
Fullness:	MEAL TOTALS		
SNACK ____ A.M./P.M.			
Hunger:			
Fullness:	MEAL TOTALS		
LUNCH ____ A.M./P.M.			
Hunger:			
Fullness:	MEAL TOTALS		
SNACK ____ A.M./P.M.			
Hunger:			
Fullness:	MEAL TOTALS		
DINNER ____ A.M./P.M.			
Hunger:			
Fullness:	MEAL TOTALS		
	DAILY TOTALS		

EXERCISE NOTES
_____ minutes

DAILY WRAP-UP
Goals: Exceeded ____ Met ____ Keep Trying ____
Notes:

Success Of The Day:

FOOD FACTOID: Humans are born with a predilection for sweetness to stimulate sucking reflexes. Breast milk, which contains the sugar lactose, has a sweet flavor.

FRIDAY

SUPPLEMENTS ☐ ☐ WEIGHT ☐

Today's Goals: _____

MEAL	FOODS & BEVERAGES	FOCUS I:	FOCUS 2:
BREAKFAST ___ A.M./P.M.			
Hunger:			
Fullness:			
	MEAL TOTALS		
SNACK ___ A.M./P.M.			
Hunger:			
Fullness:			
	MEAL TOTALS		
LUNCH ___ A.M./P.M.			
Hunger:			
Fullness:			
	MEAL TOTALS		
SNACK ___ A.M./P.M.			
Hunger:			
Fullness:			
	MEAL TOTALS		
DINNER ___ A.M./P.M.			
Hunger:			
Fullness:			
	MEAL TOTALS		
	DAILY TOTALS		

EXERCISE NOTES
_____ minutes

DAILY WRAP-UP
Goals: Exceeded ___ Met ___ Keep Trying ___
Notes:

Success Of The Day:

NUTRITION TIP: To help keep your blood pressure down, use no-salt-added ketchup. You'll save 190 mg of sodium in each tablespoon.

SATURDAY

SUPPLEMENTS ☐ ☐ WEIGHT ☐

Today's Goals:

MEAL	FOODS & BEVERAGES	FOCUS 1:	FOCUS 2:
BREAKFAST ___ A.M./P.M.			
Hunger:			
Fullness:			
	MEAL TOTALS		
SNACK ___ A.M./P.M.			
Hunger:			
Fullness:			
	MEAL TOTALS		
LUNCH ___ A.M./P.M.			
Hunger:			
Fullness:			
	MEAL TOTALS		
SNACK ___ A.M./P.M.			
Hunger:			
Fullness:			
	MEAL TOTALS		
DINNER ___ A.M./P.M.			
Hunger:			
Fullness:			
	MEAL TOTALS		
	DAILY TOTALS		

EXERCISE NOTES
_____ minutes

DAILY WRAP-UP
Goals: Exceeded ___ Met ___ Keep Trying ___
Notes:

Success Of The Day:

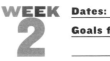

WEEK 2

Dates: _____

Goals for the Week: _____

_____

MONDAY

SUPPLEMENTS ☐ ☐   WEIGHT ☐

Today's Goals: _____

MEAL	FOODS & BEVERAGES	FOCUS I:	FOCUS 2:
BREAKFAST ____ A.M./P.M.			
Hunger:			
Fullness:			
	MEAL TOTALS		
SNACK ____ A.M./P.M.			
Hunger:			
Fullness:			
	MEAL TOTALS		
LUNCH ____ A.M./P.M.			
Hunger:			
Fullness:			
	MEAL TOTALS		
SNACK ____ A.M./P.M.			
Hunger:			
Fullness:			
	MEAL TOTALS		
DINNER ____ A.M./P.M.			
Hunger:			
Fullness:			
	MEAL TOTALS		
	DAILY TOTALS		

EXERCISE NOTES
_____ minutes

DAILY WRAP-UP
Goals: Exceeded ____ Met ____ Keep Trying ____
Notes:

Success Of The Day:

RESEARCH REPORT: In a fast-food study, subjects who ate small meals underestimated the calories by 8 percent. Those who really indulged undershot by 38 percent, guessing that their 1,188-calorie meals contained only 675 calories.

TUESDAY

SUPPLEMENTS ☐ ☐   WEIGHT ☐

Today's Goals:

MEAL	FOODS & BEVERAGES	FOCUS 1:	FOCUS 2:
BREAKFAST ____ A.M./P.M.			
Hunger:			
Fullness:			
	MEAL TOTALS		
SNACK ____ A.M./P.M.			
Hunger:			
Fullness:			
	MEAL TOTALS		
LUNCH ____ A.M./P.M.			
Hunger:			
Fullness:			
	MEAL TOTALS		
SNACK ____ A.M./P.M.			
Hunger:			
Fullness:			
	MEAL TOTALS		
DINNER ____ A.M./P.M.			
Hunger:			
Fullness:			
	MEAL TOTALS		
	DAILY TOTALS		

EXERCISE NOTES
_____ minutes

DAILY WRAP-UP
Goals: Exceeded ___ Met ___ Keep Trying ___
Notes:

Success Of The Day:

FOOD FACTOID: Frozen fruits and veggies are just as nutritious as fresh. In fact, because frozen produce is picked at its peak, it can be higher in vitamins than fresh produce shipped from afar.

FRIDAY

SUPPLEMENTS ☐ ☐   WEIGHT ☐

Today's Goals:

MEAL	FOODS & BEVERAGES	FOCUS I:	FOCUS 2:
BREAKFAST ___ A.M./P.M.			
Hunger:			
Fullness:			
	MEAL TOTALS		
SNACK ___ A.M./P.M.			
Hunger:			
Fullness:			
	MEAL TOTALS		
LUNCH ___ A.M./P.M.			
Hunger:			
Fullness:			
	MEAL TOTALS		
SNACK ___ A.M./P.M.			
Hunger:			
Fullness:			
	MEAL TOTALS		
DINNER ___ A.M./P.M.			
Hunger:			
Fullness:			
	MEAL TOTALS		
	DAILY TOTALS		

EXERCISE NOTES
_____ minutes

DAILY WRAP-UP
Goals: Exceeded ___ Met ___ Keep Trying ___
Notes:

Success Of The Day:

NUTRITION TIP: Most fruit-flavored yogurts have little or no fruit but plenty of added sugar. Try adding fresh, canned, no-sugar-added fruit to plain yogurt.

SATURDAY

SUPPLEMENTS ☐ ☐   WEIGHT ☐

Today's Goals:

MEAL	FOODS & BEVERAGES	FOCUS 1:	FOCUS 2:
BREAKFAST ____ A.M./P.M. Hunger: Fullness:			
	MEAL TOTALS		
SNACK ____ A.M./P.M. Hunger: Fullness:			
	MEAL TOTALS		
LUNCH ____ A.M./P.M. Hunger: Fullness:			
	MEAL TOTALS		
SNACK ____ A.M./P.M. Hunger: Fullness:			
	MEAL TOTALS		
DINNER ____ A.M./P.M. Hunger: Fullness:			
	MEAL TOTALS		
	DAILY TOTALS		

EXERCISE NOTES
_____ minutes

DAILY WRAP-UP
Goals: Exceeded ___   Met ___   Keep Trying ___
Notes:

Success Of The Day:

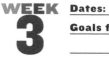

WEEK 3

Dates: _____

Goals for the Week: _____

_____

MONDAY

SUPPLEMENTS ☐ ☐   WEIGHT ☐

Today's Goals: _____

MEAL	FOODS & BEVERAGES	FOCUS I:	FOCUS 2:
BREAKFAST ____ A.M./P.M.			
Hunger:			
Fullness:			
	MEAL TOTALS		
SNACK ____ A.M./P.M.			
Hunger:			
Fullness:			
	MEAL TOTALS		
LUNCH ____ A.M./P.M.			
Hunger:			
Fullness:			
	MEAL TOTALS		
SNACK ____ A.M./P.M.			
Hunger:			
Fullness:			
	MEAL TOTALS		
DINNER ____ A.M./P.M.			
Hunger:			
Fullness:			
	MEAL TOTALS		
	DAILY TOTALS		

EXERCISE NOTES
_____ minutes

DAILY WRAP-UP
Goals: Exceeded ___ Met ___ Keep Trying ___
Notes:

Success Of The Day:

RESEARCH REPORT: Fiber in breads, cereals, and other grains may cut the risk of diabetes. In one study, researchers found a 30 percent lower risk of diabetes in people who reported eating 17 grams per day compared to those who averaged 7 grams a day.

TUESDAY

SUPPLEMENTS ☐ ☐ WEIGHT ☐

Today's Goals:

MEAL	FOODS & BEVERAGES	FOCUS 1:	FOCUS 2:
BREAKFAST ____ A.M./P.M.			
Hunger:			
Fullness:			
	MEAL TOTALS		
SNACK ____ A.M./P.M.			
Hunger:			
Fullness:			
	MEAL TOTALS		
LUNCH ____ A.M./P.M.			
Hunger:			
Fullness:			
	MEAL TOTALS		
SNACK ____ A.M./P.M.			
Hunger:			
Fullness:			
	MEAL TOTALS		
DINNER ____ A.M./P.M.			
Hunger:			
Fullness:			
	MEAL TOTALS		
	DAILY TOTALS		

EXERCISE NOTES
_____ minutes

DAILY WRAP-UP
Goals: Exceeded ____ Met ____ Keep Trying ____
Notes:
Success Of The Day:

FOOD FACTOID: Though brown-shelled eggs often cost more than eggs with white shells, they have the same nutritional content. The color of an eggshell is purely a cosmetic feature.

FRIDAY

SUPPLEMENTS ☐ ☐   WEIGHT ☐

Today's Goals:

MEAL	FOODS & BEVERAGES	FOCUS 1:	FOCUS 2:
BREAKFAST ___ A.M./P.M.			
Hunger:			
Fullness:			
	MEAL TOTALS		
SNACK ___ A.M./P.M.			
Hunger:			
Fullness:			
	MEAL TOTALS		
LUNCH ___ A.M./P.M.			
Hunger:			
Fullness:			
	MEAL TOTALS		
SNACK ___ A.M./P.M.			
Hunger:			
Fullness:			
	MEAL TOTALS		
DINNER ___ A.M./P.M.			
Hunger:			
Fullness:			
	MEAL TOTALS		
	DAILY TOTALS		

EXERCISE NOTES
_____ minutes

DAILY WRAP-UP
Goals: Exceeded ___ Met ___ Keep Trying ___
Notes:

Success Of The Day:

NUTRITION TIP: To minimize spending and maximize taste, buy produce in season. Enjoy asparagus in April, apricots in June, blueberries in July, and pears in November.

SATURDAY

SUPPLEMENTS ☐ ☐   WEIGHT ☐

Today's Goals: _____

MEAL	FOODS & BEVERAGES	FOCUS 1:	FOCUS 2:
BREAKFAST _____ A.M./P.M.			
Hunger:			
Fullness:			
	MEAL TOTALS		
SNACK _____ A.M./P.M.			
Hunger:			
Fullness:			
	MEAL TOTALS		
LUNCH _____ A.M./P.M.			
Hunger:			
Fullness:			
	MEAL TOTALS		
SNACK _____ A.M./P.M.			
Hunger:			
Fullness:			
	MEAL TOTALS		
DINNER _____ A.M./P.M.			
Hunger:			
Fullness:			
	MEAL TOTALS		
	DAILY TOTALS		

EXERCISE NOTES
_____ minutes

DAILY WRAP-UP
Goals: Exceeded ___ Met ___ Keep Trying ___
Notes:

Success Of The Day:

FITNESS FACTOID: Setting your daily exercise goal in terms of steps, rather than miles or minutes, can help with motivation. In one study, women instructed to take 10,000 steps per day averaged 10,159 steps, whereas those told to take a 30-minute walk accumulated 8,270 steps.

SUNDAY

SUPPLEMENTS ☐ ☐   WEIGHT ☐

Today's Goals:

MEAL	FOODS & BEVERAGES	FOCUS 1:	FOCUS 2:
BREAKFAST ___ A.M./P.M.			
Hunger:			
Fullness:			
	MEAL TOTALS		
SNACK ___ A.M./P.M.			
Hunger:			
Fullness:			
	MEAL TOTALS		
LUNCH ___ A.M./P.M.			
Hunger:			
Fullness:			
	MEAL TOTALS		
SNACK ___ A.M./P.M.			
Hunger:			
Fullness:			
	MEAL TOTALS		
DINNER ___ A.M./P.M.			
Hunger:			
Fullness:			
	MEAL TOTALS		
	DAILY TOTALS		

EXERCISE NOTES
_____ minutes

DAILY WRAP-UP
Goals: Exceeded ___ Met ___ Keep Trying ___
Notes:

Success Of The Day:

> "The biggest seller is cookbooks and the second is diet books — how not to eat what you've just learned how to cook."
> — ANDY ROONEY

WEEKLY WRAP-UP

SUCCESS OF THE WEEK

GOALS ASSESSMENT

EXERCISE NOTES　　　　**TOTAL DAYS EXERCISED** ☐　　**TOTAL MINUTES/ HOURS** ☐

PROGRESS REPORT

WHAT WENT WELL, AND WHY?

WHAT DIDN'T GO WELL? WHAT GOT IN MY WAY?

WHAT IS THE MOST IMPORTANT INSIGHT I GAINED ABOUT MYSELF THIS WEEK?

WHAT DO I PLAN TO DO DIFFERENTLY NEXT WEEK?

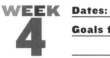

WEEK 4

Dates: _____

Goals for the Week: _____

_____

MONDAY

SUPPLEMENTS [ ] [ ]   **WEIGHT** [ ]

Today's Goals: _____

MEAL	FOODS & BEVERAGES	FOCUS 1:	FOCUS 2:
BREAKFAST ____ A.M./P.M.			
Hunger:			
Fullness:			
	MEAL TOTALS		
SNACK ____ A.M./P.M.			
Hunger:			
Fullness:			
	MEAL TOTALS		
LUNCH ____ A.M./P.M.			
Hunger:			
Fullness:			
	MEAL TOTALS		
SNACK ____ A.M./P.M.			
Hunger:			
Fullness:			
	MEAL TOTALS		
DINNER ____ A.M./P.M.			
Hunger:			
Fullness:			
	MEAL TOTALS		
	DAILY TOTALS		

EXERCISE NOTES
_____ minutes

DAILY WRAP-UP
Goals: Exceeded ___ Met ___ Keep Trying ___
Notes:

Success Of The Day:

RESEARCH REPORT: The shape of your beverage glasses influences how much you pour and drink. Whether it's beer or orange juice, studies show people pour 25 to 30 percent more into short, wide glasses than tall, skinny ones.

TUESDAY

SUPPLEMENTS ☐ ☐   WEIGHT ☐

Today's Goals:

MEAL	FOODS & BEVERAGES	FOCUS 1:	FOCUS 2:
BREAKFAST ___ A.M./P.M.			
Hunger:			
Fullness:	MEAL TOTALS		
SNACK ___ A.M./P.M.			
Hunger:			
Fullness:	MEAL TOTALS		
LUNCH ___ A.M./P.M.			
Hunger:			
Fullness:	MEAL TOTALS		
SNACK ___ A.M./P.M.			
Hunger:			
Fullness:	MEAL TOTALS		
DINNER ___ A.M./P.M.			
Hunger:			
Fullness:	MEAL TOTALS		
	DAILY TOTALS		

EXERCISE NOTES
_____ minutes

DAILY WRAP-UP
Goals: Exceeded ___ Met ___ Keep Trying ___
Notes:

Success Of The Day:

NUTRITION SHOCKER: An average-size cookie is now 7 times the size of what the **USDA** defines as a cookie serving.

WEDNESDAY

SUPPLEMENTS ☐ ☐   WEIGHT ☐

Today's Goals: _____

MEAL	FOODS & BEVERAGES	FOCUS I:	FOCUS 2:
BREAKFAST ___ A.M./P.M.			
Hunger:			
Fullness:	MEAL TOTALS		
SNACK ___ A.M./P.M.			
Hunger:			
Fullness:	MEAL TOTALS		
LUNCH ___ A.M./P.M.			
Hunger:			
Fullness:	MEAL TOTALS		
SNACK ___ A.M./P.M.			
Hunger:			
Fullness:	MEAL TOTALS		
DINNER ___ A.M./P.M.			
Hunger:			
Fullness:	MEAL TOTALS		
	DAILY TOTALS		

EXERCISE NOTES
_____ minutes

DAILY WRAP-UP
Goals: Exceeded ___ Met ___ Keep Trying ___
Notes:

Success Of The Day:

BY THE NUMBERS: **246:** Dollars, in millions, that Coca-Cola spent to promote Coke products in 2004. **3:** Dollars, in millions, the U.S. government spent in a year on the Five A Day for Better Health campaign in support of fruits and vegetables.

THURSDAY

SUPPLEMENTS ☐ ☐   WEIGHT ☐

Today's Goals:

MEAL	FOODS & BEVERAGES	FOCUS I:	FOCUS 2:
BREAKFAST ___ A.M./P.M.			
Hunger:			
Fullness:			
	MEAL TOTALS		
SNACK ___ A.M./P.M.			
Hunger:			
Fullness:			
	MEAL TOTALS		
LUNCH ___ A.M./P.M.			
Hunger:			
Fullness:			
	MEAL TOTALS		
SNACK ___ A.M./P.M.			
Hunger:			
Fullness:			
	MEAL TOTALS		
DINNER ___ A.M./P.M.			
Hunger:			
Fullness:			
	MEAL TOTALS		
	DAILY TOTALS		

EXERCISE NOTES
_____ minutes

DAILY WRAP-UP
Goals: Exceeded ___ Met ___ Keep Trying ___
Notes:

Success Of The Day:

FOOD FACTOID: Federal law allows most products a **20 percent** variance for the calorie counts listed on food labels, so a cookie labeled **300** calories can legally contain up to **360 calories.**

FRIDAY

SUPPLEMENTS ☐ ☐   WEIGHT ☐

Today's Goals: _____

MEAL	FOODS & BEVERAGES	FOCUS I:	FOCUS 2:
BREAKFAST ___ A.M./P.M.			
Hunger:			
Fullness:	MEAL TOTALS		
SNACK ___ A.M./P.M.			
Hunger:			
Fullness:	MEAL TOTALS		
LUNCH ___ A.M./P.M.			
Hunger:			
Fullness:	MEAL TOTALS		
SNACK ___ A.M./P.M.			
Hunger:			
Fullness:	MEAL TOTALS		
DINNER ___ A.M./P.M.			
Hunger:			
Fullness:	MEAL TOTALS		
	DAILY TOTALS		

EXERCISE NOTES
_____ minutes

DAILY WRAP-UP
Goals: Exceeded ___ Met ___ Keep Trying ___
Notes:

Success Of The Day:

NUTRITION TIP: By buying generic food brands, you can save as much as 50 percent on items from pasta sauce to cereal to salad dressing. With name brands, much of the money goes into advertising and packaging.

SATURDAY

SUPPLEMENTS ☐☐   WEIGHT ☐

Today's Goals:

MEAL	FOODS & BEVERAGES	FOCUS 1:	FOCUS 2:
BREAKFAST ____ A.M./P.M.			
Hunger:			
Fullness:			
	MEAL TOTALS		
SNACK ____ A.M./P.M.			
Hunger:			
Fullness:			
	MEAL TOTALS		
LUNCH ____ A.M./P.M.			
Hunger:			
Fullness:			
	MEAL TOTALS		
SNACK ____ A.M./P.M.			
Hunger:			
Fullness:			
	MEAL TOTALS		
DINNER ____ A.M./P.M.			
Hunger:			
Fullness:			
	MEAL TOTALS		
	DAILY TOTALS		

EXERCISE NOTES
_____ minutes

DAILY WRAP-UP
Goals: Exceeded ____ Met ____ Keep Trying ____
Notes:

Success Of The Day:

FITNESS FACTOID: Studies suggest that yoga and meditation can alter your brain, helping you live a calmer life and possibly increasing your immune function. Not only do you feel refreshed after each session, but the sense of calm and happiness builds over time.

SUNDAY

SUPPLEMENTS ☐ ☐   WEIGHT ☐

Today's Goals:

MEAL	FOODS & BEVERAGES	FOCUS 1:	FOCUS 2:
BREAKFAST ____ A.M./P.M.			
Hunger:			
Fullness:			
	MEAL TOTALS		
SNACK ____ A.M./P.M.			
Hunger:			
Fullness:			
	MEAL TOTALS		
LUNCH ____ A.M./P.M.			
Hunger:			
Fullness:			
	MEAL TOTALS		
SNACK ____ A.M./P.M.			
Hunger:			
Fullness:			
	MEAL TOTALS		
DINNER ____ A.M./P.M.			
Hunger:			
Fullness:			
	MEAL TOTALS		
	DAILY TOTALS		

EXERCISE NOTES
_____ minutes

DAILY WRAP-UP
Goals: Exceeded ____ Met ____ Keep Trying ____
Notes:

Success Of The Day:

"One cannot think well, love well, sleep well, if one has not dined well."

—VIRGINIA WOOLF

WEEKLY WRAP-UP

SUCCESS OF THE WEEK

GOALS ASSESSMENT

EXERCISE NOTES	**TOTAL DAYS EXERCISED**	**TOTAL MINUTES/ HOURS**	

PROGRESS REPORT

WHAT WENT WELL, AND WHY?

WHAT DIDN'T GO WELL? WHAT GOT IN MY WAY?

WHAT IS THE MOST IMPORTANT INSIGHT I GAINED ABOUT MYSELF THIS WEEK?

WHAT DO I PLAN TO DO DIFFERENTLY NEXT WEEK?

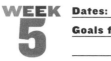

WEEK 5

MONDAY

SUPPLEMENTS ☐ ☐   WEIGHT ☐

Today's Goals: _____

MEAL	FOODS & BEVERAGES	FOCUS I:	FOCUS 2:
BREAKFAST ___ A.M./P.M.			
Hunger:			
Fullness:			
	MEAL TOTALS		
SNACK ___ A.M./P.M.			
Hunger:			
Fullness:			
	MEAL TOTALS		
LUNCH ___ A.M./P.M.			
Hunger:			
Fullness:			
	MEAL TOTALS		
SNACK ___ A.M./P.M.			
Hunger:			
Fullness:			
	MEAL TOTALS		
DINNER ___ A.M./P.M.			
Hunger:			
Fullness:			
	MEAL TOTALS		
	DAILY TOTALS		

EXERCISE NOTES
_____ minutes

DAILY WRAP-UP
Goals: Exceeded ___ Met ___ Keep Trying ___
Notes:

Success Of The Day:

RESEARCH REPORT: Eating a large, 100-calorie salad as a first course may reduce the calories you eat in the entire meal by as much as 12 percent, compared to not eating salad. However, eating a 400-calorie salad may increase your total calorie intake by 17 percent.

TUESDAY

SUPPLEMENTS ☐ ☐ WEIGHT ☐

Today's Goals:

MEAL	FOODS & BEVERAGES	FOCUS 1:	FOCUS 2:
BREAKFAST ___ A.M./P.M.			
Hunger:			
Fullness:			
	MEAL TOTALS		
SNACK ___ A.M./P.M.			
Hunger:			
Fullness:			
	MEAL TOTALS		
LUNCH ___ A.M./P.M.			
Hunger:			
Fullness:			
	MEAL TOTALS		
SNACK ___ A.M./P.M.			
Hunger:			
Fullness:			
	MEAL TOTALS		
DINNER ___ A.M./P.M.			
Hunger:			
Fullness:			
	MEAL TOTALS		
	DAILY TOTALS		

EXERCISE NOTES
_____ minutes

DAILY WRAP-UP
Goals: Exceeded ___ Met ___ Keep Trying ___
Notes:

Success Of The Day:

NUTRITION SHOCKER: One Reuben sandwich contains 3,270 mg of sodium, far more than the 2,300 mg maximum recommended per day. One Dunkin' Donuts salt bagel contains 4,520 mg of sodium.

WEDNESDAY

SUPPLEMENTS ☐ ☐   WEIGHT ☐

Today's Goals:

MEAL	FOODS & BEVERAGES	FOCUS 1:	FOCUS 2:
BREAKFAST ____ A.M./P.M.			
Hunger:			
Fullness:			
	MEAL TOTALS		
SNACK ____ A.M./P.M.			
Hunger:			
Fullness:			
	MEAL TOTALS		
LUNCH ____ A.M./P.M.			
Hunger:			
Fullness:			
	MEAL TOTALS		
SNACK ____ A.M./P.M.			
Hunger:			
Fullness:			
	MEAL TOTALS		
DINNER ____ A.M./P.M.			
Hunger:			
Fullness:			
	MEAL TOTALS		
	DAILY TOTALS		

EXERCISE NOTES
_____ minutes

DAILY WRAP-UP
Goals: Exceeded ____   Met ____   Keep Trying ____
Notes:

Success Of The Day:

BY THE NUMBERS: 6: Number of weeks humans can survive without food. **7:** Number of days we can survive without water, our most important nutrient.

THURSDAY

SUPPLEMENTS ☐ ☐   WEIGHT ☐

Today's Goals:

MEAL	FOODS & BEVERAGES	FOCUS I:	FOCUS 2:
BREAKFAST ___ A.M./P.M.			
Hunger:			
Fullness:			
	MEAL TOTALS		
SNACK ___ A.M./P.M.			
Hunger:			
Fullness:			
	MEAL TOTALS		
LUNCH ___ A.M./P.M.			
Hunger:			
Fullness:			
	MEAL TOTALS		
SNACK ___ A.M./P.M.			
Hunger:			
Fullness:			
	MEAL TOTALS		
DINNER ___ A.M./P.M.			
Hunger:			
Fullness:			
	MEAL TOTALS		
	DAILY TOTALS		

EXERCISE NOTES
_____ minutes

DAILY WRAP-UP
Goals: Exceeded ___ Met ___ Keep Trying ___
Notes:

Success Of The Day:

FOOD FACTOID: The terms "enriched" and "fortified" aren't synonymous. "Enriched" means nutrients lost during processing have been added back in. "Fortified" indicates that nutrients not originally present have been added, such as vitamin D in milk.

FRIDAY

SUPPLEMENTS ☐ ☐   WEIGHT ☐

Today's Goals:

MEAL	FOODS & BEVERAGES	FOCUS I:	FOCUS 2:
BREAKFAST ___ A.M./P.M.			
Hunger:			
Fullness:			
	MEAL TOTALS		
SNACK ___ A.M./P.M.			
Hunger:			
Fullness:			
	MEAL TOTALS		
LUNCH ___ A.M./P.M.			
Hunger:			
Fullness:			
	MEAL TOTALS		
SNACK ___ A.M./P.M.			
Hunger:			
Fullness:			
	MEAL TOTALS		
DINNER ___ A.M./P.M.			
Hunger:			
Fullness:			
	MEAL TOTALS		
	DAILY TOTALS		

EXERCISE NOTES
_____ minutes

DAILY WRAP-UP
Goals: Exceeded ___ Met ___ Keep Trying ___
Notes:

Success Of The Day:

NUTRITION TIP: To save time, make nutritious foods in double batches. Grill extra vegetables and refrigerate them for use later as a pizza topping, omelet filler, or sandwich layer. Use the black beans from tonight's chili for tomorrow's salad or soup.

SATURDAY

SUPPLEMENTS ☐ ☐ WEIGHT ☐

Today's Goals:

MEAL	FOODS & BEVERAGES	FOCUS 1:	FOCUS 2:
BREAKFAST ___ A.M./P.M.			
Hunger:			
Fullness:	MEAL TOTALS		
SNACK ___ A.M./P.M.			
Hunger:			
Fullness:	MEAL TOTALS		
LUNCH A.M./P.M.			
Hunger:			
Fullness:	MEAL TOTALS		
SNACK ___ A.M./P.M.			
Hunger:			
Fullness:	MEAL TOTALS		
DINNER ___ A.M./P.M.			
Hunger:			
Fullness:	MEAL TOTALS		
	DAILY TOTALS		

EXERCISE NOTES
_____ minutes

DAILY WRAP-UP
Goals: Exceeded ___ Met ___ Keep Trying ___
Notes:

Success Of The Day:

FITNESS FACTOID: Crunches performed on a stability ball challenge the abdominal muscles much more than a traditional crunch done on the floor. One study found that the ball was most effective when positioned under the lower lumbar region of the spine.

SUNDAY

SUPPLEMENTS ☐ ☐   WEIGHT ☐

Today's Goals:

MEAL	FOODS & BEVERAGES	FOCUS I:	FOCUS 2:
BREAKFAST ____ A.M./P.M.			
Hunger:			
Fullness:	MEAL TOTALS		
SNACK ____ A.M./P.M.			
Hunger:			
Fullness:	MEAL TOTALS		
LUNCH ____ A.M./P.M.			
Hunger:			
Fullness:	MEAL TOTALS		
SNACK ____ A.M./P.M.			
Hunger:			
Fullness:	MEAL TOTALS		
DINNER ____ A.M./P.M.			
Hunger:			
Fullness:	MEAL TOTALS		
	DAILY TOTALS		

EXERCISE NOTES
_____ minutes

DAILY WRAP-UP
Goals: Exceeded ____   Met ____   Keep Trying ____
Notes:

Success Of The Day:

"An optimist is a person who starts a new diet on Thanksgiving Day."
— IRV KUPCINET, talk-show host

WEEKLY WRAP-UP

SUCCESS OF THE WEEK

GOALS ASSESSMENT

EXERCISE NOTES	**TOTAL DAYS EXERCISED**		**TOTAL MINUTES/ HOURS**	

PROGRESS REPORT

WHAT WENT WELL, AND WHY?

WHAT DIDN'T GO WELL? WHAT GOT IN MY WAY?

WHAT IS THE MOST IMPORTANT INSIGHT I GAINED ABOUT MYSELF THIS WEEK?

WHAT DO I PLAN TO DO DIFFERENTLY NEXT WEEK?

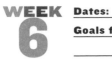

WEEK 6

Dates: _____

Goals for the Week: _____

_____

MONDAY

SUPPLEMENTS ☐ ☐ WEIGHT ☐

Today's Goals: _____

MEAL	FOODS & BEVERAGES	FOCUS I:	FOCUS 2:
BREAKFAST ___ A.M./P.M.			
Hunger:			
Fullness:			
	MEAL TOTALS		
SNACK ___ A.M./P.M.			
Hunger:			
Fullness:			
	MEAL TOTALS		
LUNCH ___ A.M./P.M.			
Hunger:			
Fullness:			
	MEAL TOTALS		
SNACK ___ A.M./P.M.			
Hunger:			
Fullness:			
	MEAL TOTALS		
DINNER ___ A.M./P.M.			
Hunger:			
Fullness:			
	MEAL TOTALS		
	DAILY TOTALS		

EXERCISE NOTES
_____ minutes

DAILY WRAP-UP
Goals: Exceeded ___ Met ___ Keep Trying ___
Notes:

Success Of The Day:

RESEARCH REPORT: It's never too late to adopt healthy habits. In one study, adults ages 45 to 64 who started eating five fruits and veggies daily and exercising 2.5 hours per week and who maintained a BMI of 30 or less reduced their death rate 40 percent compared to people with less healthy lifestyles.

TUESDAY

SUPPLEMENTS ☐ ☐ WEIGHT ☐

Today's Goals:

MEAL	FOODS & BEVERAGES	FOCUS I:	FOCUS 2:
BREAKFAST ___ A.M./P.M.			
Hunger:			
Fullness:			
	MEAL TOTALS		
SNACK ___ A.M./P.M.			
Hunger:			
Fullness:			
	MEAL TOTALS		
LUNCH ___ A.M./P.M.			
Hunger:			
Fullness:			
	MEAL TOTALS		
SNACK ___ A.M./P.M.			
Hunger:			
Fullness:			
	MEAL TOTALS		
DINNER ___ A.M./P.M.			
Hunger:			
Fullness:			
	MEAL TOTALS		
	DAILY TOTALS		

EXERCISE NOTES
_____ minutes

DAILY WRAP-UP
Goals: Exceeded ___ Met ___ Keep Trying ___
Notes:

Success Of The Day:

FOOD FACTOID: Just because a food package features a picture of a fruit doesn't mean there's any of that particular fruit in the product. Those chewy bits of fruit in some brands of "strawberries and cream" instant oatmeal are actually dehydrated apples dyed red.

FRIDAY

SUPPLEMENTS ☐ ☐   WEIGHT ☐

Today's Goals:

MEAL	FOODS & BEVERAGES	FOCUS 1:	FOCUS 2:
BREAKFAST ___ A.M./P.M.			
Hunger:			
Fullness:	MEAL TOTALS		
SNACK ___ A.M./P.M.			
Hunger:			
Fullness:	MEAL TOTALS		
LUNCH ___ A.M./P.M.			
Hunger:			
Fullness:	MEAL TOTALS		
SNACK ___ A.M./P.M.			
Hunger:			
Fullness:	MEAL TOTALS		
DINNER ___ A.M./P.M.			
Hunger:			
Fullness:	MEAL TOTALS		
	DAILY TOTALS		

EXERCISE NOTES
_____ minutes

DAILY WRAP-UP
Goals: Exceeded ___   Met ___   Keep Trying ___
Notes:

Success Of The Day:

NUTRITION TIP: When assembling your dinner plate, try this visual: half your plate should be veggies, one-quarter should be whole grains, and one-quarter should be protein.

SATURDAY

SUPPLEMENTS ☐ ☐   WEIGHT ☐

Today's Goals: _____

MEAL	FOODS & BEVERAGES	FOCUS I:	FOCUS 2:
BREAKFAST ____ A.M./P.M.			
Hunger:			
Fullness:			
	MEAL TOTALS		
SNACK ____ A.M./P.M.			
Hunger:			
Fullness:			
	MEAL TOTALS		
LUNCH ____ A.M./P.M.			
Hunger:			
Fullness:			
	MEAL TOTALS		
SNACK ____ A.M./P.M.			
Hunger:			
Fullness:			
	MEAL TOTALS		
DINNER ____ A.M./P.M.			
Hunger:			
Fullness:			
	MEAL TOTALS		
	DAILY TOTALS		

EXERCISE NOTES
_____ minutes

DAILY WRAP-UP
Goals: Exceeded ____ Met ____ Keep Trying ____
Notes:

Success Of The Day:

FITNESS FACTOID: Strength training can turn back the clock. In one study, postmenopausal women who lifted weights twice a week for a year had the strength and bone-density levels of women 15 to 20 years younger.

SUNDAY

SUPPLEMENTS ☐ ☐   WEIGHT ☐

Today's Goals:

MEAL	FOODS & BEVERAGES	FOCUS 1:	FOCUS 2:
BREAKFAST ____ A.M./P.M.			
Hunger:			
Fullness:	MEAL TOTALS		
SNACK ____ A.M./P.M.			
Hunger:			
Fullness:	MEAL TOTALS		
LUNCH ____ A.M./P.M.			
Hunger:			
Fullness:	MEAL TOTALS		
SNACK ____ A.M./P.M.			
Hunger:			
Fullness:	MEAL TOTALS		
DINNER ____ A.M./P.M.			
Hunger:			
Fullness:	MEAL TOTALS		
	DAILY TOTALS		

EXERCISE NOTES
_____ minutes

DAILY WRAP-UP
Goals: Exceeded ____ Met ____ Keep Trying ____
Notes:

Success Of The Day:

"When I buy cookies, I eat just four and throw the rest away. But first I spray them with Raid so I won't dig them out of the garbage later. Be careful, though, because Raid really doesn't taste that bad."
— JANETTE BARBER, stand-up comic

WEEKLY WRAP-UP

SUCCESS OF THE WEEK

GOALS ASSESSMENT

EXERCISE NOTES	**TOTAL DAYS EXERCISED**		**TOTAL MINUTES/ HOURS**	

PROGRESS REPORT

WHAT WENT WELL, AND WHY?

WHAT DIDN'T GO WELL? WHAT GOT IN MY WAY?

WHAT IS THE MOST IMPORTANT INSIGHT I GAINED ABOUT MYSELF THIS WEEK?

WHAT DO I PLAN TO DO DIFFERENTLY NEXT WEEK?

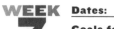 **WEEK 7**

Dates: _____

Goals for the Week: _____

_____

MONDAY

SUPPLEMENTS [   ] [   ]   WEIGHT [   ]

Today's Goals: _____

MEAL	FOODS & BEVERAGES	FOCUS I:	FOCUS 2:
BREAKFAST ___ A.M./P.M.			
Hunger:			
Fullness:			
	MEAL TOTALS		
SNACK ___ A.M./P.M.			
Hunger:			
Fullness:			
	MEAL TOTALS		
LUNCH ___ A.M./P.M.			
Hunger:			
Fullness:			
	MEAL TOTALS		
SNACK ___ A.M./P.M.			
Hunger:			
Fullness:			
	MEAL TOTALS		
DINNER ___ A.M./P.M.			
Hunger:			
Fullness:			
	MEAL TOTALS		
	DAILY TOTALS		

EXERCISE NOTES
_____ minutes

DAILY WRAP-UP
Goals: Exceeded ___   Met ___   Keep Trying ___
Notes:

Success Of The Day:

RESEARCH REPORT: If you eat with one other person, you'll eat 35 percent more than you would eating alone, 75 percent more if you're at a table for four. If you eat with a group of seven or more — think Thanksgiving dinner — you'll scarf down 96 percent more calories.

TUESDAY

SUPPLEMENTS ☐ ☐   WEIGHT ☐

Today's Goals:

MEAL	FOODS & BEVERAGES	FOCUS 1:	FOCUS 2:
BREAKFAST ___ A.M./P.M.			
Hunger:			
Fullness:			
	MEAL TOTALS		
SNACK ___ A.M./P.M.			
Hunger:			
Fullness:			
	MEAL TOTALS		
LUNCH ___ A.M./P.M.			
Hunger:			
Fullness:			
	MEAL TOTALS		
SNACK ___ A.M./P.M.			
Hunger:			
Fullness:			
	MEAL TOTALS		
DINNER ___ A.M./P.M.			
Hunger:			
Fullness:			
	MEAL TOTALS		
	DAILY TOTALS		

EXERCISE NOTES
_____ minutes

DAILY WRAP-UP
Goals: Exceeded ___ Met ___ Keep Trying ___
Notes:

Success Of The Day:

NUTRITION SHOCKER: Worldwide, the number of people who eat too much has surpassed the number of people afflicted by hunger.

WEDNESDAY

SUPPLEMENTS ☐ ☐ WEIGHT ☐

Today's Goals:

MEAL	FOODS & BEVERAGES	FOCUS 1:	FOCUS 2:
BREAKFAST ___ A.M./P.M.			
Hunger:			
Fullness:	MEAL TOTALS		
SNACK ___ A.M./P.M.			
Hunger:			
Fullness:	MEAL TOTALS		
LUNCH ___ A.M./P.M.			
Hunger:			
Fullness:	MEAL TOTALS		
SNACK ___ A.M./P.M.			
Hunger:			
Fullness:	MEAL TOTALS		
DINNER ___ A.M./P.M.			
Hunger:			
Fullness:	MEAL TOTALS		
	DAILY TOTALS		

EXERCISE NOTES
_____ minutes

DAILY WRAP-UP
Goals: Exceeded ___ Met ___ Keep Trying ___
Notes:

Success Of The Day:

BY THE NUMBERS: 75: Percent of our sodium intake that comes from processed foods. **5 to 10:** Percent we get from table salt and cooking salt. **10:** Percent occurring naturally in food. **150,000:** Lives that could be saved annually by a 50 percent reduction of sodium in packaged and restaurant foods.

THURSDAY

SUPPLEMENTS ☐ ☐   WEIGHT ☐

Today's Goals:

MEAL	FOODS & BEVERAGES	FOCUS I:	FOCUS 2:
BREAKFAST ___ A.M./P.M.			
Hunger:			
Fullness:	MEAL TOTALS		
SNACK ___ A.M./P.M.			
Hunger:			
Fullness:	MEAL TOTALS		
LUNCH ___ A.M./P.M.			
Hunger:			
Fullness:	MEAL TOTALS		
SNACK ___ A.M./P.M.			
Hunger:			
Fullness:	MEAL TOTALS		
DINNER ___ A.M./P.M.			
Hunger:			
Fullness:	MEAL TOTALS		
	DAILY TOTALS		

EXERCISE NOTES
_____ minutes

DAILY WRAP-UP
Goals: Exceeded ___ Met ___ Keep Trying ___
Notes:

Success Of The Day:

FOOD FACTOID: Carotenoids, pigments found in colorful fruits and veggies, may help prevent heart disease and cancer and boost immunity. Rich sources include carrots, sweet potatoes, broccoli, collard greens, mangoes, pineapple, peaches, and oranges.

FRIDAY

SUPPLEMENTS ☐ ☐　WEIGHT ☐

Today's Goals:

MEAL	FOODS & BEVERAGES	FOCUS I:	FOCUS 2:
BREAKFAST ___ A.M./P.M.			
Hunger:			
Fullness:			
	MEAL TOTALS		
SNACK ___ A.M./P.M.			
Hunger:			
Fullness:			
	MEAL TOTALS		
LUNCH ___ A.M./P.M.			
Hunger:			
Fullness:			
	MEAL TOTALS		
SNACK ___ A.M./P.M.			
Hunger:			
Fullness:			
	MEAL TOTALS		
DINNER ___ A.M./P.M.			
Hunger:			
Fullness:			
	MEAL TOTALS		
	DAILY TOTALS		

EXERCISE NOTES
_____ minutes

DAILY WRAP-UP
Goals: Exceeded ___　Met ___　Keep Trying ___
Notes:

Success Of The Day:

NUTRITION TIP: To save calories, choose foods whose volume comes largely from air, water, or fiber. Examples include a pint of grape tomatoes (60 calories), 4 cups of air-popped popcorn (120 calories), and 1 cup of sweet red bell pepper strips (70 calories).

SATURDAY

SUPPLEMENTS ☐ ☐ WEIGHT ☐

Today's Goals:

MEAL	FOODS & BEVERAGES	FOCUS 1:	FOCUS 2:
BREAKFAST ___ A.M./P.M.			
Hunger:			
Fullness:	MEAL TOTALS		
SNACK ___ A.M./P.M.			
Hunger:			
Fullness:	MEAL TOTALS		
LUNCH ___ A.M./P.M.			
Hunger:			
Fullness:	MEAL TOTALS		
SNACK ___ A.M./P.M.			
Hunger:			
Fullness:	MEAL TOTALS		
DINNER ___ A.M./P.M.			
Hunger:			
Fullness:	MEAL TOTALS		
	DAILY TOTALS		

EXERCISE NOTES
_____ minutes

DAILY WRAP-UP
Goals: Exceeded ___ Met ___ Keep Trying ___
Notes:

Success Of The Day:

FITNESS FACTOID: Compared to inactive moms-to-be, women who exercise during pregnancy have a lower risk of gestational diabetes and high blood pressure, experience fewer aches and pains, gain on average 7 pounds less, deliver leaner babies, and recuperate more quickly.

SUNDAY

SUPPLEMENTS ☐ ☐ WEIGHT ☐

Today's Goals:

MEAL	FOODS & BEVERAGES	FOCUS I:	FOCUS 2:
BREAKFAST ___ A.M./P.M.			
Hunger:			
Fullness:			
	MEAL TOTALS		
SNACK ___ A.M./P.M.			
Hunger:			
Fullness:			
	MEAL TOTALS		
LUNCH ___ A.M./P.M.			
Hunger:			
Fullness:			
	MEAL TOTALS		
SNACK ___ A.M./P.M.			
Hunger:			
Fullness:			
	MEAL TOTALS		
DINNER ___ A.M./P.M.			
Hunger:			
Fullness:			
	MEAL TOTALS		
	DAILY TOTALS		

EXERCISE NOTES
_____ minutes

DAILY WRAP-UP
Goals: Exceeded ___ Met ___ Keep Trying ___
Notes:

Success Of The Day:

"I keep trying to lose weight . . . but it keeps finding me!"

— ANONYMOUS

WEEKLY WRAP-UP

SUCCESS OF THE WEEK

GOALS ASSESSMENT

EXERCISE NOTES   **TOTAL DAYS EXERCISED**   **TOTAL MINUTES/ HOURS**

PROGRESS REPORT

WHAT WENT WELL, AND WHY?

WHAT DIDN'T GO WELL? WHAT GOT IN MY WAY?

WHAT IS THE MOST IMPORTANT INSIGHT I GAINED ABOUT MYSELF THIS WEEK?

WHAT DO I PLAN TO DO DIFFERENTLY NEXT WEEK?

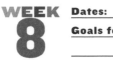

WEEK 8

Dates: _____

Goals for the Week: _____

_____

MONDAY

SUPPLEMENTS ☐ ☐   WEIGHT ☐

Today's Goals: _____

MEAL	FOODS & BEVERAGES	FOCUS I:	FOCUS 2:
BREAKFAST ____ A.M./P.M.			
Hunger:			
Fullness:	MEAL TOTALS		
SNACK ____ A.M./P.M.			
Hunger:			
Fullness:	MEAL TOTALS		
LUNCH ____ A.M./P.M.			
Hunger:			
Fullness:	MEAL TOTALS		
SNACK ____ A.M./P.M.			
Hunger:			
Fullness:	MEAL TOTALS		
DINNER ____ A.M./P.M.			
Hunger:			
Fullness:	MEAL TOTALS		
	DAILY TOTALS		

EXERCISE NOTES
_____ minutes

DAILY WRAP-UP
Goals: Exceeded ____ Met ____ Keep Trying ____
Notes:

Success Of The Day:

RESEARCH REPORT: Large dishes, bowls, and serving utensils skew your idea of what's a normal serving and prompt you to eat more — as much as 57 percent more when it comes to large ice cream bowls and scoops and 53 percent more with jumbo bowls of Chex Mix.

TUESDAY

SUPPLEMENTS ☐ ☐ WEIGHT ☐

Today's Goals:

MEAL	FOODS & BEVERAGES	FOCUS I:	FOCUS 2:
BREAKFAST ___ A.M./P.M.			
Hunger:			
Fullness:			
	MEAL TOTALS		
SNACK ___ A.M./P.M.			
Hunger:			
Fullness:			
	MEAL TOTALS		
LUNCH ___ A.M./P.M.			
Hunger:			
Fullness:			
	MEAL TOTALS		
SNACK ___ A.M./P.M.			
Hunger:			
Fullness:			
	MEAL TOTALS		
DINNER ___ A.M./P.M.			
Hunger:			
Fullness:			
	MEAL TOTALS		
	DAILY TOTALS		

EXERCISE NOTES
_____ minutes

DAILY WRAP-UP
Goals: Exceeded ___ Met ___ Keep Trying ___
Notes:

Success Of The Day:

FOOD FACTOID: Soft drinks are the number one source of calories in teens' diets and the only individual food directly linked to obesity.

FRIDAY

SUPPLEMENTS [ ] [ ]   WEIGHT [ ]

Today's Goals: _____

MEAL	FOODS & BEVERAGES	FOCUS I:	FOCUS 2:
BREAKFAST ___ A.M./P.M. Hunger: Fullness:			
	MEAL TOTALS		
SNACK ___ A.M./P.M. Hunger: Fullness:			
	MEAL TOTALS		
LUNCH ___ A.M./P.M. Hunger: Fullness:			
	MEAL TOTALS		
SNACK ___ A.M./P.M. Hunger: Fullness:			
	MEAL TOTALS		
DINNER ___ A.M./P.M. Hunger: Fullness:			
	MEAL TOTALS		
	DAILY TOTALS		

EXERCISE NOTES
_____ minutes

DAILY WRAP-UP
Goals: Exceeded ___ Met ___ Keep Trying ___
Notes:

Success Of The Day:

NUTRITION TIP: When purchasing breads, cereals, and other grain items, follow this rule: buy only products with at least 3 grams of fiber per serving.

SATURDAY

SUPPLEMENTS ☐ ☐   WEIGHT ☐

Today's Goals: _____

MEAL	FOODS & BEVERAGES	FOCUS 1:	FOCUS 2:
BREAKFAST ___ A.M./P.M.			
Hunger:			
Fullness:			
	MEAL TOTALS		
SNACK ___ A.M./P.M.			
Hunger:			
Fullness:			
	MEAL TOTALS		
LUNCH ___ A.M./P.M.			
Hunger:			
Fullness:			
	MEAL TOTALS		
SNACK ___ A.M./P.M.			
Hunger:			
Fullness:			
	MEAL TOTALS		
DINNER ___ A.M./P.M.			
Hunger:			
Fullness:			
	MEAL TOTALS		
	DAILY TOTALS		

EXERCISE NOTES
_____ minutes

DAILY WRAP-UP
Goals: Exceeded ___ Met ___ Keep Trying ___
Notes:

Success Of The Day:

FITNESS FACTOID: You're never too old or overweight to benefit from exercise. Working out just 3 days a week for 75 minutes total can improve the fitness of postmenopausal women who are overweight and inactive, research suggests. With more fitness comes less heart disease.

SUNDAY

SUPPLEMENTS ☐ ☐   WEIGHT ☐

Today's Goals: _____

MEAL	FOODS & BEVERAGES	FOCUS I:	FOCUS 2:
BREAKFAST ____ A.M./P.M.			
Hunger:			
Fullness:	MEAL TOTALS		
SNACK ____ A.M./P.M.			
Hunger:			
Fullness:	MEAL TOTALS		
LUNCH ____ A.M./P.M.			
Hunger:			
Fullness:	MEAL TOTALS		
SNACK ____ A.M./P.M.			
Hunger:			
Fullness:	MEAL TOTALS		
DINNER ____ A.M./P.M.			
Hunger:			
Fullness:	MEAL TOTALS		
	DAILY TOTALS		

EXERCISE NOTES
_____ minutes

DAILY WRAP-UP
Goals: Exceeded ___ Met ___ Keep Trying ___
Notes:

Success Of The Day:

"It's difficult to think anything but pleasant thoughts while eating a homegrown tomato." — LEWIS GRIZZARD

WEEKLY WRAP-UP

SUCCESS OF THE WEEK

GOALS ASSESSMENT

EXERCISE NOTES   TOTAL DAYS EXERCISED [ ]   TOTAL MINUTES/ HOURS [ ]

PROGRESS REPORT

WHAT WENT WELL, AND WHY?

WHAT DIDN'T GO WELL? WHAT GOT IN MY WAY?

WHAT IS THE MOST IMPORTANT INSIGHT I GAINED ABOUT MYSELF THIS WEEK?

WHAT DO I PLAN TO DO DIFFERENTLY NEXT WEEK?

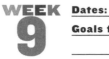

WEEK 9

Dates: _____

Goals for the Week: _____

_____

MONDAY

SUPPLEMENTS ☐ ☐ WEIGHT ☐

Today's Goals: _____

MEAL	FOODS & BEVERAGES	FOCUS I:	FOCUS 2:
BREAKFAST ___ A.M./P.M.			
Hunger:			
Fullness:	MEAL TOTALS		
SNACK ___ A.M./P.M.			
Hunger:			
Fullness:	MEAL TOTALS		
LUNCH ___ A.M./P.M.			
Hunger:			
Fullness:	MEAL TOTALS		
SNACK ___ A.M./P.M.			
Hunger:			
Fullness:	MEAL TOTALS		
DINNER ___ A.M./P.M.			
Hunger:			
Fullness:	MEAL TOTALS		
	DAILY TOTALS		

EXERCISE NOTES
_____ minutes

DAILY WRAP-UP
Goals: Exceeded ___ Met ___ Keep Trying ___
Notes:
Success Of The Day:

RESEARCH REPORT: Compared to men who watch TV an hour or less per week, men who tuned in for 2 to 10 hours per week had a 66 percent greater diabetes risk. Men who watched 21 to 40 hours had twice the risk.

TUESDAY

SUPPLEMENTS ☐ ☐ WEIGHT ☐

Today's Goals:

MEAL	FOODS & BEVERAGES	FOCUS 1:	FOCUS 2:
BREAKFAST ___ A.M./P.M.			
Hunger:			
Fullness:	MEAL TOTALS		
SNACK ___ A.M./P.M.			
Hunger:			
Fullness:	MEAL TOTALS		
LUNCH ___ A.M./P.M.			
Hunger:			
Fullness:	MEAL TOTALS		
SNACK ___ A.M./P.M.			
Hunger:			
Fullness:	MEAL TOTALS		
DINNER ___ A.M./P.M.			
Hunger:			
Fullness:	MEAL TOTALS		
	DAILY TOTALS		

EXERCISE NOTES
_____ minutes

DAILY WRAP-UP
Goals: Exceeded ___ Met ___ Keep Trying ___
Notes:

Success Of The Day:

NUTRITION SHOCKER: The latest edition of <u>Joy of Cooking</u> contains the same brownie recipe as the original, but the new edition makes 16 brownies instead of 30, which means the portions are twice as large.

WEDNESDAY   SUPPLEMENTS ☐☐   WEIGHT ☐

Today's Goals:

MEAL	FOODS & BEVERAGES	FOCUS I:	FOCUS 2:
BREAKFAST ___ A.M./P.M.			
Hunger:			
Fullness:	MEAL TOTALS		
SNACK ___ A.M./P.M.			
Hunger:			
Fullness:	MEAL TOTALS		
LUNCH ___ A.M./P.M.			
Hunger:			
Fullness:	MEAL TOTALS		
SNACK ___ A.M./P.M.			
Hunger:			
Fullness:	MEAL TOTALS		
DINNER ___ A.M./P.M.			
Hunger:			
Fullness:	MEAL TOTALS		
	DAILY TOTALS		

EXERCISE NOTES
_____ minutes

DAILY WRAP-UP
Goals: Exceeded ___ Met ___ Keep Trying ___
Notes:

Success Of The Day:

BY THE NUMBERS: **70:** Percentage of supermarket shoppers who bring shopping lists into the store. **10:** Percentage of shoppers who stick to their lists. **2:** Number of additional items that shoppers pick up for each item on their list.

THURSDAY

SUPPLEMENTS ☐ ☐   WEIGHT ☐

Today's Goals:

MEAL	FOODS & BEVERAGES	FOCUS 1:	FOCUS 2:
BREAKFAST ____ A.M./P.M.			
Hunger:			
Fullness:			
	MEAL TOTALS		
SNACK ____ A.M./P.M.			
Hunger:			
Fullness:			
	MEAL TOTALS		
LUNCH ____ A.M./P.M.			
Hunger:			
Fullness:			
	MEAL TOTALS		
SNACK ____ A.M./P.M.			
Hunger:			
Fullness:			
	MEAL TOTALS		
DINNER ____ A.M./P.M.			
Hunger:			
Fullness:			
	MEAL TOTALS		
	DAILY TOTALS		

EXERCISE NOTES
_____ minutes

DAILY WRAP-UP
Goals: Exceeded ___ Met ___ Keep Trying ___
Notes:

Success Of The Day:

FOOD FACTOID: It's not true that calories you eat after 7 P.M. turn to fat. If you eat more calories than you burn, no matter what the clock says, you'll gain fat. If you eat fewer calories than you burn — even if some are consumed during The Tonight Show — you'll slim down.

FRIDAY

SUPPLEMENTS ☐ ☐ WEIGHT ☐

Today's Goals: _____

MEAL	FOODS & BEVERAGES	FOCUS I:	FOCUS 2:
BREAKFAST ___ A.M./P.M.			
Hunger:			
Fullness:			
	MEAL TOTALS		
SNACK ___ A.M./P.M.			
Hunger:			
Fullness:			
	MEAL TOTALS		
LUNCH ___ A.M./P.M.			
Hunger:			
Fullness:			
	MEAL TOTALS		
SNACK ___ A.M./P.M.			
Hunger:			
Fullness:			
	MEAL TOTALS		
DINNER ___ A.M./P.M.			
Hunger:			
Fullness:			
	MEAL TOTALS		
	DAILY TOTALS		

EXERCISE NOTES
_____ minutes

DAILY WRAP-UP
Goals: Exceeded ___ Met ___ Keep Trying ___
Notes:

Success Of The Day:

NUTRITION TIP: You'll eat more of whatever you buy in bulk, so save bulk purchases at discount stores for nutritious staples such as rice, lentils, beans, tuna, frozen fish, and chicken breasts.

SATURDAY

SUPPLEMENTS ☐ ☐ WEIGHT ☐

Today's Goals:

MEAL	FOODS & BEVERAGES	FOCUS 1:	FOCUS 2:
BREAKFAST ___ A.M./P.M.			
Hunger:			
Fullness:			
	MEAL TOTALS		
SNACK ___ A.M./P.M.			
Hunger:			
Fullness:			
	MEAL TOTALS		
LUNCH ___ A.M./P.M.			
Hunger:			
Fullness:			
	MEAL TOTALS		
SNACK ___ A.M./P.M.			
Hunger:			
Fullness:			
	MEAL TOTALS		
DINNER ___ A.M./P.M.			
Hunger:			
Fullness:			
	MEAL TOTALS		
	DAILY TOTALS		

EXERCISE NOTES
_____ minutes

DAILY WRAP-UP
Goals: Exceeded ___ Met ___ Keep Trying ___
Notes:

Success Of The Day:

FITNESS FACTOID: Exercise can help keep your brain in tip-top shape. In one study, adults who walked 3 times a week for 45 minutes performed significantly better on decision-making tests than inactive people.

SUNDAY

SUPPLEMENTS ☐ ☐   WEIGHT ☐

Today's Goals:

MEAL	FOODS & BEVERAGES	FOCUS I:	FOCUS 2:
BREAKFAST ___ A.M./P.M.			
Hunger:			
Fullness:	MEAL TOTALS		
SNACK ___ A.M./P.M.			
Hunger:			
Fullness:	MEAL TOTALS		
LUNCH ___ A.M./P.M.			
Hunger:			
Fullness:	MEAL TOTALS		
SNACK ___ A.M./P.M.			
Hunger:			
Fullness:	MEAL TOTALS		
DINNER ___ A.M./P.M.			
Hunger:			
Fullness:	MEAL TOTALS		
	DAILY TOTALS		

EXERCISE NOTES
_____ minutes

DAILY WRAP-UP
Goals: Exceeded ___   Met ___   Keep Trying ___
Notes:

Success Of The Day:

"Eating a vegetarian diet, exercising every day, and meditating is considered radical. Allowing someone to slice your chest open and graft your leg veins in your heart is considered normal and conservative." — DEAN ORNISH

WEEKLY WRAP-UP

SUCCESS OF THE WEEK

GOALS ASSESSMENT

EXERCISE NOTES   TOTAL DAYS EXERCISED [   ]   TOTAL MINUTES/ HOURS [   ]

PROGRESS REPORT

WHAT WENT WELL, AND WHY?

WHAT DIDN'T GO WELL? WHAT GOT IN MY WAY?

WHAT IS THE MOST IMPORTANT INSIGHT I GAINED ABOUT MYSELF THIS WEEK?

WHAT DO I PLAN TO DO DIFFERENTLY NEXT WEEK?

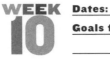

WEEK 10

Dates: _____

Goals for the Week: _____

_____

MONDAY

SUPPLEMENTS ☐ ☐   WEIGHT ☐

Today's Goals: _____

MEAL	FOODS & BEVERAGES	FOCUS 1:	FOCUS 2:
BREAKFAST ____ A.M./P.M.			
Hunger:			
Fullness:			
	MEAL TOTALS		
SNACK ____ A.M./P.M.			
Hunger:			
Fullness:			
	MEAL TOTALS		
LUNCH ____ A.M./P.M.			
Hunger:			
Fullness:			
	MEAL TOTALS		
SNACK ____ A.M./P.M.			
Hunger:			
Fullness:			
	MEAL TOTALS		
DINNER ____ A.M./P.M.			
Hunger:			
Fullness:			
	MEAL TOTALS		
	DAILY TOTALS		

EXERCISE NOTES
_____ minutes

DAILY WRAP-UP
Goals: Exceeded ____ Met ____ Keep Trying ____
Notes:
Success Of The Day:

RESEARCH REPORT: The intense sweetness in diet beverages may contribute to conditioning for a high preference for sweetness, some studies suggest. So while diet sodas are a better choice than sugar-sweetened sodas, unsweetened drinks like water and tea are best.

TUESDAY

SUPPLEMENTS [ ] [ ]   WEIGHT [ ]

Today's Goals:

MEAL	FOODS & BEVERAGES	FOCUS 1:	FOCUS 2:
BREAKFAST ___ A.M./P.M.			
Hunger:			
Fullness:			
	MEAL TOTALS		
SNACK ___ A.M./P.M.			
Hunger:			
Fullness:			
	MEAL TOTALS		
LUNCH ___ A.M./P.M.			
Hunger:			
Fullness:			
	MEAL TOTALS		
SNACK ___ A.M./P.M.			
Hunger:			
Fullness:			
	MEAL TOTALS		
DINNER ___ A.M./P.M.			
Hunger:			
Fullness:			
	MEAL TOTALS		
	DAILY TOTALS		

EXERCISE NOTES
_____ minutes

DAILY WRAP-UP
Goals: Exceeded ___ Met ___ Keep Trying ___
Notes:

Success Of The Day:

FOOD FACTOID: Alcohol not only stimulates appetite but also loosens your inhibitions, so you may be less careful about your food choices. Lowest-calorie choice: light beer, which contains about 100 calories per 12 ounces.

FRIDAY

SUPPLEMENTS ☐ ☐   WEIGHT ☐

Today's Goals:

MEAL	FOODS & BEVERAGES	FOCUS 1:	FOCUS 2:
BREAKFAST ____ A.M./P.M.			
Hunger:			
Fullness:			
	MEAL TOTALS		
SNACK ____ A.M./P.M.			
Hunger:			
Fullness:			
	MEAL TOTALS		
LUNCH ____ A.M./P.M.			
Hunger:			
Fullness:			
	MEAL TOTALS		
SNACK ____ A.M./P.M.			
Hunger:			
Fullness:			
	MEAL TOTALS		
DINNER ____ A.M./P.M.			
Hunger:			
Fullness:			
	MEAL TOTALS		
	DAILY TOTALS		

EXERCISE NOTES
_____ minutes

DAILY WRAP-UP
Goals: Exceeded ____ Met ____ Keep Trying ____
Notes:

Success Of The Day:

NUTRITION TIP: Arrive at the supermarket with a full stomach and a shopping list set in stone so that you avoid buying junk food on impulse.

SATURDAY

SUPPLEMENTS ☐ ☐   WEIGHT ☐

Today's Goals:

MEAL	FOODS & BEVERAGES	FOCUS I:	FOCUS 2:
BREAKFAST ____ A.M./P.M.			
Hunger:			
Fullness:			
	MEAL TOTALS		
SNACK ____ A.M./P.M.			
Hunger:			
Fullness:			
	MEAL TOTALS		
LUNCH ____ A.M./P.M.			
Hunger:			
Fullness:			
	MEAL TOTALS		
SNACK ____ A.M./P.M.			
Hunger:			
Fullness:			
	MEAL TOTALS		
DINNER ____ A.M./P.M.			
Hunger:			
Fullness:			
	MEAL TOTALS		
	DAILY TOTALS		

EXERCISE NOTES
_____ minutes

DAILY WRAP-UP
Goals: Exceeded ____ Met ____ Keep Trying ____
Notes:

Success Of The Day:

FITNESS FACTOID: Though your resting heart rate is partly genetically determined, as you gain fitness, this number drops. A couch potato's heart may have to work twice as hard — **80 beats per minute** compared to **40 bpm** — to pump the same blood volume as a top athlete's.

SUNDAY

SUPPLEMENTS ☐ ☐   WEIGHT ☐

Today's Goals:

MEAL	FOODS & BEVERAGES	FOCUS 1:	FOCUS 2:
BREAKFAST ___ A.M./P.M.			
Hunger:			
Fullness:			
	MEAL TOTALS		
SNACK ___ A.M./P.M.			
Hunger:			
Fullness:			
	MEAL TOTALS		
LUNCH ___ A.M./P.M.			
Hunger:			
Fullness:			
	MEAL TOTALS		
SNACK ___ A.M./P.M.			
Hunger:			
Fullness:			
	MEAL TOTALS		
DINNER ___ A.M./P.M.			
Hunger:			
Fullness:			
	MEAL TOTALS		
	DAILY TOTALS		

EXERCISE NOTES
_____ minutes

DAILY WRAP-UP
Goals: Exceeded ___ Met ___ Keep Trying ___
Notes:

Success Of The Day:

"Laughter is brightest where food is best." — IRISH PROVERB

WEEKLY WRAP-UP

SUCCESS OF THE WEEK

GOALS ASSESSMENT

EXERCISE NOTES   **TOTAL DAYS EXERCISED** [ ]   **TOTAL MINUTES/ HOURS** [ ]

PROGRESS REPORT

WHAT WENT WELL, AND WHY?

WHAT DIDN'T GO WELL? WHAT GOT IN MY WAY?

WHAT IS THE MOST IMPORTANT INSIGHT I GAINED ABOUT MYSELF THIS WEEK?

WHAT DO I PLAN TO DO DIFFERENTLY NEXT WEEK?

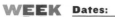

WEEK 11

Dates: _____

Goals for the Week: _____

_____

MONDAY

SUPPLEMENTS ☐ ☐   WEIGHT ☐

Today's Goals: _____

MEAL	FOODS & BEVERAGES		FOCUS I:	FOCUS 2:
BREAKFAST ____ A.M./P.M.				
Hunger:				
Fullness:				
	MEAL TOTALS			
SNACK ____ A.M./P.M.				
Hunger:				
Fullness:				
	MEAL TOTALS			
LUNCH ____ A.M./P.M.				
Hunger:				
Fullness:				
	MEAL TOTALS			
SNACK ____ A.M./P.M.				
Hunger:				
Fullness:				
	MEAL TOTALS			
DINNER ____ A.M./P.M.				
Hunger:				
Fullness:				
	MEAL TOTALS			
	DAILY TOTALS			

EXERCISE NOTES
_____ minutes

DAILY WRAP-UP
Goals: Exceeded ___ Met ___ Keep Trying ___
Notes:

Success Of The Day:

RESEARCH REPORT: Lack of sleep impacts hormones that regulate appetite, increasing obesity risk. In one study, adults who slept 6 hours a night were 23 percent more likely to be obese than those who slept 7 to 9 hours. Those averaging 5 hours were 50 percent more likely to be obese.

TUESDAY

SUPPLEMENTS ☐ ☐   WEIGHT ☐

Today's Goals:

MEAL	FOODS & BEVERAGES	FOCUS 1:	FOCUS 2:
BREAKFAST ____ A.M./P.M.			
Hunger:			
Fullness:	MEAL TOTALS		
SNACK ____ A.M./P.M.			
Hunger:			
Fullness:	MEAL TOTALS		
LUNCH ____ A.M./P.M.			
Hunger:			
Fullness:	MEAL TOTALS		
SNACK ____ A.M./P.M.			
Hunger:			
Fullness:	MEAL TOTALS		
DINNER ____ A.M./P.M.			
Hunger:			
Fullness:	MEAL TOTALS		
	DAILY TOTALS		

EXERCISE NOTES
_____ minutes

DAILY WRAP-UP
Goals: Exceeded ____   Met ____   Keep Trying ____
Notes:

Success Of The Day:

FOOD FACTOID: "No-calorie" cooking-oil sprays aren't actually calorie-free. The government defines a serving size as a spray lasting $\frac{1}{4}$ second, which contains $\frac{1}{4}$ gram of fat, but on food labels, servings containing less than $\frac{1}{2}$ gram needn't be listed. A l-second spray contains 9 calories.

FRIDAY

SUPPLEMENTS ☐ ☐ WEIGHT ☐

Today's Goals:

MEAL	FOODS & BEVERAGES	FOCUS I:	FOCUS 2:
BREAKFAST ___ A.M./P.M.			
Hunger:			
Fullness:			
	MEAL TOTALS		
SNACK ___ A.M./P.M.			
Hunger:			
Fullness:			
	MEAL TOTALS		
LUNCH ___ A.M./P.M.			
Hunger:			
Fullness:			
	MEAL TOTALS		
SNACK ___ A.M./P.M.			
Hunger:			
Fullness:			
	MEAL TOTALS		
DINNER ___ A.M./P.M.			
Hunger:			
Fullness:			
	MEAL TOTALS		
	DAILY TOTALS		

EXERCISE NOTES
_____ minutes

DAILY WRAP-UP
Goals: Exceeded ___ Met ___ Keep Trying ___
Notes:

Success Of The Day:

NUTRITION TIP: You can eliminate 40 percent of the sodium in canned veggies by pouring off the brine from the can and rinsing the vegetables.

SATURDAY

SUPPLEMENTS ☐ ☐   WEIGHT ☐

Today's Goals:

MEAL	FOODS & BEVERAGES	FOCUS I:	FOCUS 2:
BREAKFAST ___ A.M./P.M.			
Hunger:			
Fullness:			
	MEAL TOTALS		
SNACK ___ A.M./P.M.			
Hunger:			
Fullness:			
	MEAL TOTALS		
LUNCH ___ A.M./P.M.			
Hunger:			
Fullness:			
	MEAL TOTALS		
SNACK ___ A.M./P.M.			
Hunger:			
Fullness:			
	MEAL TOTALS		
DINNER ___ A.M./P.M.			
Hunger:			
Fullness:			
	MEAL TOTALS		
	DAILY TOTALS		

EXERCISE NOTES
_____ minutes

DAILY WRAP-UP
Goals: Exceeded ___ Met ___ Keep Trying ___
Notes:

Success Of The Day:

FITNESS FACTOID: An hour of moderate exercise, accumulated throughout the day, can lower your diabetes risk by nearly 50 percent, primarily by controlling weight and allowing your body to make better use of its insulin.

SUNDAY

SUPPLEMENTS ☐ ☐   WEIGHT ☐

Today's Goals:

MEAL	FOODS & BEVERAGES	FOCUS I:	FOCUS 2:
BREAKFAST ___ A.M./P.M.			
Hunger: Fullness:			
	MEAL TOTALS		
SNACK ___ A.M./P.M.			
Hunger: Fullness:			
	MEAL TOTALS		
LUNCH ___ A.M./P.M.			
Hunger: Fullness:			
	MEAL TOTALS		
SNACK ___ A.M./P.M.			
Hunger: Fullness:			
	MEAL TOTALS		
DINNER ___ A.M./P.M.			
Hunger: Fullness:			
	MEAL TOTALS		
	DAILY TOTALS		

EXERCISE NOTES
_____ minutes

DAILY WRAP-UP
Goals: Exceeded ___ Met ___ Keep Trying ___
Notes:

Success Of The Day:

"The bagel, an unsweetened doughnut with rigor mortis."
— BEATRICE **and** IRA FREEMAN

WEEKLY WRAP-UP

SUCCESS OF THE WEEK

GOALS ASSESSMENT

EXERCISE NOTES | TOTAL DAYS EXERCISED | | TOTAL MINUTES/ HOURS |

PROGRESS REPORT

WHAT WENT WELL, AND WHY?

WHAT DIDN'T GO WELL? WHAT GOT IN MY WAY?

WHAT IS THE MOST IMPORTANT INSIGHT I GAINED ABOUT MYSELF THIS WEEK?

WHAT DO I PLAN TO DO DIFFERENTLY NEXT WEEK?

WEEK 12

Dates: _____

Goals for the Week: _____

_____

MONDAY

SUPPLEMENTS [ ] [ ]   WEIGHT [ ]

Today's Goals: _____

MEAL	FOODS & BEVERAGES	FOCUS 1:	FOCUS 2:
BREAKFAST ____ A.M./P.M.			
Hunger:			
Fullness:			
	MEAL TOTALS		
SNACK ____ A.M./P.M.			
Hunger:			
Fullness:			
	MEAL TOTALS		
LUNCH ____ A.M./P.M.			
Hunger:			
Fullness:			
	MEAL TOTALS		
SNACK ____ A.M./P.M.			
Hunger:			
Fullness:			
	MEAL TOTALS		
DINNER ____ A.M./P.M.			
Hunger:			
Fullness:			
	MEAL TOTALS		
	DAILY TOTALS		

EXERCISE NOTES
_____ minutes

DAILY WRAP-UP
Goals: Exceeded ____ Met ____ Keep Trying ____

Notes:

Success Of The Day:

RESEARCH REPORT: Adding a little fat can give you a lot more nutrition. When lettuce, carrots, or spinach were eaten with avocado, test subjects absorbed 8 to 13 times more antioxidants, including beta carotene, linked to cancer and heart disease reduction.

TUESDAY

SUPPLEMENTS ☐ ☐   WEIGHT ☐

Today's Goals: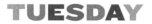

MEAL	FOODS & BEVERAGES	FOCUS I:	FOCUS 2:
BREAKFAST _____ A.M./P.M. Hunger: Fullness:			
	MEAL TOTALS		
SNACK _____ A.M./P.M. Hunger: Fullness:			
	MEAL TOTALS		
LUNCH _____ A.M./P.M. Hunger: Fullness:			
	MEAL TOTALS		
SNACK _____ A.M./P.M. Hunger: Fullness:			
	MEAL TOTALS		
DINNER _____ A.M./P.M. Hunger: Fullness:			
	MEAL TOTALS		
	DAILY TOTALS		

EXERCISE NOTES
_____ minutes

DAILY WRAP-UP
Goals: Exceeded ___ Met ___ Keep Trying ___
Notes:

Success Of The Day:

FOOD FACTOID: Vitamin C isn't the only nutrient that prevents colds. Vitamin A, including its plant form beta carotene, helps form the membranes inside your nose and mouth, which in turn form the protective barrier that keeps bacteria and viruses from invading.

FRIDAY

SUPPLEMENTS ☐ ☐   WEIGHT ☐

Today's Goals:

MEAL	FOODS & BEVERAGES	FOCUS 1:	FOCUS 2:
BREAKFAST ____ A.M./P.M.			
Hunger:			
Fullness:			
	MEAL TOTALS		
SNACK ____ A.M./P.M.			
Hunger:			
Fullness:			
	MEAL TOTALS		
LUNCH ____ A.M./P.M.			
Hunger:			
Fullness:			
	MEAL TOTALS		
SNACK ____ A.M./P.M.			
Hunger:			
Fullness:			
	MEAL TOTALS		
DINNER ____ A.M./P.M.			
Hunger:			
Fullness:			
	MEAL TOTALS		
	DAILY TOTALS		

EXERCISE NOTES
_____ minutes

DAILY WRAP-UP
Goals: Exceeded ____ Met ____ Keep Trying ____
Notes:

Success Of The Day:

NUTRITION TIP: Family-style meals lead to overeating, so everyone in your family should put their food on their plate before sitting down to eat. It's fine to keep salad or fruit on the table.

SATURDAY

SUPPLEMENTS ☐ ☐ WEIGHT ☐

Today's Goals:

MEAL	FOODS & BEVERAGES	FOCUS I:	FOCUS 2:
BREAKFAST _____ A.M./P.M.			
Hunger: Fullness:			
	MEAL TOTALS		
SNACK _____ A.M./P.M.			
Hunger: Fullness:			
	MEAL TOTALS		
LUNCH _____ A.M./P.M.			
Hunger: Fullness:			
	MEAL TOTALS		
SNACK _____ A.M./P.M.			
Hunger: Fullness:			
	MEAL TOTALS		
DINNER _____ A.M./P.M.			
Hunger: Fullness:			
	MEAL TOTALS		
	DAILY TOTALS		

EXERCISE NOTES
_____ minutes

DAILY WRAP-UP
Goals: Exceeded ___ Met ___ Keep Trying ___
Notes:

Success Of The Day:

FITNESS FACTOID: Walking just 30 minutes a day is enough to increase bone density, according to a review of 24 studies. Compared to sedentary women, those who took up walking for at least 4 months showed a 2 percent increase in bone density.

SUNDAY

SUPPLEMENTS ☐ ☐ WEIGHT ☐

Today's Goals:

MEAL	FOODS & BEVERAGES	FOCUS I:	FOCUS 2:
BREAKFAST ___ A.M./P.M.			
Hunger:			
Fullness:			
	MEAL TOTALS		
SNACK ___ A.M./P.M.			
Hunger:			
Fullness:			
	MEAL TOTALS		
LUNCH ___ A.M./P.M.			
Hunger:			
Fullness:			
	MEAL TOTALS		
SNACK ___ A.M./P.M.			
Hunger:			
Fullness:			
	MEAL TOTALS		
DINNER ___ A.M./P.M.			
Hunger:			
Fullness:			
	MEAL TOTALS		
	DAILY TOTALS		

EXERCISE NOTES
_____ minutes

DAILY WRAP-UP
Goals: Exceeded ___ Met ___ Keep Trying ___
Notes:

Success Of The Day:

"People are so worried about what they eat between Christmas and the New Year, but they really should be worried about what they eat between the New Year and Christmas." — AUTHOR UNKNOWN

WEEKLY WRAP-UP

SUCCESS OF THE WEEK

GOALS ASSESSMENT

EXERCISE NOTES　　　　　**TOTAL DAYS EXERCISED**　　　　**TOTAL MINUTES/ HOURS**

PROGRESS REPORT

WHAT WENT WELL, AND WHY?

WHAT DIDN'T GO WELL? WHAT GOT IN MY WAY?

WHAT IS THE MOST IMPORTANT INSIGHT I GAINED ABOUT MYSELF THIS WEEK?

WHAT DO I PLAN TO DO DIFFERENTLY NEXT WEEK?

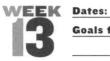

WEEK 13

MONDAY

SUPPLEMENTS ☐ ☐   WEIGHT ☐

Today's Goals: _____

MEAL	FOODS & BEVERAGES	FOCUS I:	FOCUS 2:
BREAKFAST ____ A.M./P.M.			
Hunger:			
Fullness:			
	MEAL TOTALS		
SNACK ____ A.M./P.M.			
Hunger:			
Fullness:			
	MEAL TOTALS		
LUNCH ____ A.M./P.M.			
Hunger:			
Fullness:			
	MEAL TOTALS		
SNACK ____ A.M./P.M.			
Hunger:			
Fullness:			
	MEAL TOTALS		
DINNER ____ A.M./P.M.			
Hunger:			
Fullness:			
	MEAL TOTALS		
	DAILY TOTALS		

EXERCISE NOTES
_____ minutes

DAILY WRAP-UP
Goals: Exceeded ____ Met ____ Keep Trying ____
Notes:

Success Of The Day:

RESEARCH REPORT: Your lifestyle can dramatically reduce your cancer risk. Thirty percent to 40 percent of all cancers — 420,000 to 560,000 cases per year — are caused by poor eating habits, excess weight, and inactivity, according to the American Institute for Cancer Research.

TUESDAY

SUPPLEMENTS ☐ ☐   WEIGHT ☐

Today's Goals:

MEAL	FOODS & BEVERAGES	FOCUS I:	FOCUS 2:
BREAKFAST ____ A.M./P.M. Hunger: Fullness:			
	MEAL TOTALS		
SNACK ____ A.M./P.M. Hunger: Fullness:			
	MEAL TOTALS		
LUNCH ____ A.M./P.M. Hunger: Fullness:			
	MEAL TOTALS		
SNACK ____ A.M./P.M. Hunger: Fullness:			
	MEAL TOTALS		
DINNER ____ A.M./P.M. Hunger: Fullness:			
	MEAL TOTALS		
	DAILY TOTALS		

EXERCISE NOTES
_____ minutes

DAILY WRAP-UP
Goals: Exceeded ____   Met ____   Keep Trying ____
Notes:

Success Of The Day:

FOOD FACTOID: Emotional eaters typically consume 3 times more food than they would under normal circumstances. When an eating bout is triggered by emotions versus seeing or smelling food, you're less likely to take price or nutritional value into consideration.

FRI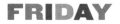DAY

SUPPLEMENTS ☐ ☐ WEIGHT ☐

Today's Goals:

MEAL	FOODS & BEVERAGES	FOCUS I:	FOCUS 2:
BREAKFAST ___ A.M./P.M.			
Hunger:			
Fullness:			
	MEAL TOTALS		
SNACK ___ A.M./P.M.			
Hunger:			
Fullness:			
	MEAL TOTALS		
LUNCH ___ A.M./P.M.			
Hunger:			
Fullness:			
	MEAL TOTALS		
SNACK ___ A.M./P.M.			
Hunger:			
Fullness:			
	MEAL TOTALS		
DINNER ___ A.M./P.M.			
Hunger:			
Fullness:			
	MEAL TOTALS		
	DAILY TOTALS		

EXERCISE NOTES
_____ minutes

DAILY WRAP-UP
Goals: Exceeded ___ Met ___ Keep Trying ___
Notes:

Success Of The Day:

NUTRITION TIP: If you don't like the taste of plain water, add a splash of 100 percent fruit juice instead of table or artificial sugar. A quarter cup of white grape or apple juice per 20 ounces adds just 30 calories and counts as a quarter of a fruit serving.

SATURDAY

SUPPLEMENTS ☐ ☐   WEIGHT ☐

Today's Goals:

MEAL	FOODS & BEVERAGES	FOCUS I:	FOCUS 2:
BREAKFAST ____ A.M./P.M.			
Hunger:			
Fullness:			
	MEAL TOTALS		
SNACK ____ A.M./P.M.			
Hunger:			
Fullness:			
	MEAL TOTALS		
LUNCH ____ A.M./P.M.			
Hunger:			
Fullness:			
	MEAL TOTALS		
SNACK ____ A.M./P.M.			
Hunger:			
Fullness:			
	MEAL TOTALS		
DINNER ____ A.M./P.M.			
Hunger:			
Fullness:			
	MEAL TOTALS		
	DAILY TOTALS		

EXERCISE NOTES
_____ minutes

DAILY WRAP-UP
Goals: Exceeded ____ Met ____ Keep Trying ____
Notes:

Success Of The Day:

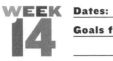

WEEK 14

Dates: _____

Goals for the Week: _____

_____

MONDAY

SUPPLEMENTS ☐ ☐   WEIGHT ☐

Today's Goals: _____

MEAL	FOODS & BEVERAGES	FOCUS I:	FOCUS 2:
BREAKFAST ____ A.M./P.M.			
Hunger:			
Fullness:	MEAL TOTALS		
SNACK ____ A.M./P.M.			
Hunger:			
Fullness:	MEAL TOTALS		
LUNCH ____ A.M./P.M.			
Hunger:			
Fullness:	MEAL TOTALS		
SNACK ____ A.M./P.M.			
Hunger:			
Fullness:	MEAL TOTALS		
DINNER ____ A.M./P.M.			
Hunger:			
Fullness:	MEAL TOTALS		
	DAILY TOTALS		

EXERCISE NOTES
_____ minutes

DAILY WRAP-UP

Goals: Exceeded ____ Met ____ Keep Trying ____

Notes:

Success Of The Day:

RESEARCH REPORT: Trans-fat consumption has been linked to infertility. An 8-year study of 18,000 married women found that infertility risk increased by 73 percent with each 2 percent increase in calories derived from trans fat.

TUESDAY

SUPPLEMENTS ☐ ☐   WEIGHT ☐

Today's Goals:

MEAL	FOODS & BEVERAGES	FOCUS 1:	FOCUS 2:
BREAKFAST ___ A.M./P.M.			
Hunger:			
Fullness:			
	MEAL TOTALS		
SNACK ___ A.M./P.M.			
Hunger:			
Fullness:			
	MEAL TOTALS		
LUNCH ___ A.M./P.M.			
Hunger:			
Fullness:			
	MEAL TOTALS		
SNACK ___ A.M./P.M.			
Hunger:			
Fullness:			
	MEAL TOTALS		
DINNER ___ A.M./P.M.			
Hunger:			
Fullness:			
	MEAL TOTALS		
	DAILY TOTALS		

EXERCISE NOTES
_____ minutes

DAILY WRAP-UP
Goals: Exceeded ___ Met ___ Keep Trying ___
Notes:

Success Of The Day:

FOOD FACTOID: Limiting meat helps the environment. Replacing one 3.5-ounce beef serving, one egg, and a 1-ounce serving of cheese daily with produce, beans, and whole grains spares the need for **40** pounds of fertilizer each year and the dumping of **11,400** pounds of animal manure.

FRIDAY

SUPPLEMENTS ☐ ☐   WEIGHT ☐

Today's Goals:

MEAL	FOODS & BEVERAGES	FOCUS 1:	FOCUS 2:
BREAKFAST ___ A.M./P.M.			
Hunger:			
Fullness:	MEAL TOTALS		
SNACK ___ A.M./P.M.			
Hunger:			
Fullness:	MEAL TOTALS		
LUNCH ___ A.M./P.M.			
Hunger:			
Fullness:	MEAL TOTALS		
SNACK ___ A.M./P.M.			
Hunger:			
Fullness:	MEAL TOTALS		
DINNER ___ A.M./P.M.			
Hunger:			
Fullness:	MEAL TOTALS		
	DAILY TOTALS		

EXERCISE NOTES
_____ minutes

DAILY WRAP-UP
Goals: Exceeded ___ Met ___ Keep Trying ___
Notes:
Success Of The Day:

NUTRITION TIP: When perusing the nutrition facts on a package, check both the serving size and the number of servings per container. A 20-ounce bottle of tea may be one serving to you, but might actually contain 2.5 servings — which means 2.5 times more calories than it seems at first glance.

SATURDAY

SUPPLEMENTS ☐ ☐   WEIGHT ☐

Today's Goals:

MEAL	FOODS & BEVERAGES	FOCUS I:	FOCUS 2:
BREAKFAST ___ A.M./P.M.			
Hunger:			
Fullness:			
	MEAL TOTALS		
SNACK ___ A.M./P.M.			
Hunger:			
Fullness:			
	MEAL TOTALS		
LUNCH ___ A.M./P.M.			
Hunger:			
Fullness:			
	MEAL TOTALS		
SNACK ___ A.M./P.M.			
Hunger:			
Fullness:			
	MEAL TOTALS		
DINNER ___ A.M./P.M.			
Hunger:			
Fullness:			
	MEAL TOTALS		
	DAILY TOTALS		

EXERCISE NOTES
_____ minutes

DAILY WRAP-UP
Goals: Exceeded ___ Met ___ Keep Trying ___
Notes:

Success Of The Day:

FITNESS FACTOID: A great way to combat workout boredom is "disassociation," aka "tuning out." Research shows that people who are able to distract themselves — whether it's watching **CNN**, listening to music, or daydreaming — enjoy their workouts more and exercise longer.

SUNDAY

SUPPLEMENTS ☐ ☐   WEIGHT ☐

Today's Goals:

MEAL	FOODS & BEVERAGES	FOCUS I:	FOCUS 2:
BREAKFAST ___ A.M./P.M.			
Hunger:			
Fullness:			
	MEAL TOTALS		
SNACK ___ A.M./P.M.			
Hunger:			
Fullness:			
	MEAL TOTALS		
LUNCH ___ A.M./P.M.			
Hunger:			
Fullness:			
	MEAL TOTALS		
SNACK ___ A.M./P.M.			
Hunger:			
Fullness:			
	MEAL TOTALS		
DINNER ___ A.M./P.M.			
Hunger:			
Fullness:			
	MEAL TOTALS		
	DAILY TOTALS		

EXERCISE NOTES
_____ minutes

DAILY WRAP-UP
Goals: Exceeded ___ Met ___ Keep Trying ___
Notes:

Success Of The Day:

"My doctor told me to stop having intimate dinners for four, unless there are three other people."
— ORSON WELLES

WEEKLY WRAP-UP

SUCCESS OF THE WEEK

GOALS ASSESSMENT

EXERCISE NOTES | TOTAL DAYS EXERCISED | TOTAL MINUTES/ HOURS

PROGRESS REPORT

WHAT WENT WELL, AND WHY?

WHAT DIDN'T GO WELL? WHAT GOT IN MY WAY?

WHAT IS THE MOST IMPORTANT INSIGHT I GAINED ABOUT MYSELF THIS WEEK?

WHAT DO I PLAN TO DO DIFFERENTLY NEXT WEEK?

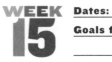

WEEK 15

MONDAY

SUPPLEMENTS ☐ ☐   WEIGHT ☐

Today's Goals: _____

MEAL	FOODS & BEVERAGES	FOCUS 1:	FOCUS 2:
BREAKFAST ____ A.M./P.M.			
Hunger:			
Fullness:			
	MEAL TOTALS		
SNACK ____ A.M./P.M.			
Hunger:			
Fullness:			
	MEAL TOTALS		
LUNCH ____ A.M./P.M.			
Hunger:			
Fullness:			
	MEAL TOTALS		
SNACK ____ A.M./P.M.			
Hunger:			
Fullness:			
	MEAL TOTALS		
DINNER ____ A.M./P.M.			
Hunger:			
Fullness:			
	MEAL TOTALS		
	DAILY TOTALS		

EXERCISE NOTES
_____ minutes

DAILY WRAP-UP
Goals: Exceeded ____ Met ____ Keep Trying ____
Notes:

Success Of The Day:

RESEARCH REPORT: The more hassle a food is to eat, the less you'll consume. When secretaries had to open a desk drawer to eat Hershey's Kisses, they ate one-third fewer Kisses than when the chocolates were right on their desks. When they had to walk 6 feet to get the Kisses, they ate even fewer.

TUESDAY

SUPPLEMENTS ☐ ☐ WEIGHT ☐

Today's Goals: _____

MEAL	FOODS & BEVERAGES	FOCUS 1:	FOCUS 2:
BREAKFAST ___ A.M./P.M.			
Hunger:			
Fullness:			
	MEAL TOTALS		
SNACK ___ A.M./P.M.			
Hunger:			
Fullness:			
	MEAL TOTALS		
LUNCH ___ A.M./P.M.			
Hunger:			
Fullness:			
	MEAL TOTALS		
SNACK ___ A.M./P.M.			
Hunger:			
Fullness:			
	MEAL TOTALS		
DINNER ___ A.M./P.M.			
Hunger:			
Fullness:			
	MEAL TOTALS		
	DAILY TOTALS		

EXERCISE NOTES
_____ minutes

DAILY WRAP-UP
Goals: Exceeded ___ Met ___ Keep Trying ___
Notes:

Success Of The Day:

NUTRITION SHOCKER: Soft drinks are the single biggest source of calories in the American diet, providing about 7 percent of calories. One of every four beverages consumed today in America is a soft drink.

WEDNESDAY   SUPPLEMENTS ☐ ☐   WEIGHT ☐

Today's Goals:

MEAL	FOODS & BEVERAGES	FOCUS I:	FOCUS 2:
BREAKFAST ____ A.M./P.M.			
Hunger:			
Fullness:			
	MEAL TOTALS		
SNACK ____ A.M./P.M.			
Hunger:			
Fullness:			
	MEAL TOTALS		
LUNCH ____ A.M./P.M.			
Hunger:			
Fullness:			
	MEAL TOTALS		
SNACK ____ A.M./P.M.			
Hunger:			
Fullness:			
	MEAL TOTALS		
DINNER ____ A.M./P.M.			
Hunger:			
Fullness:			
	MEAL TOTALS		
	DAILY TOTALS		

EXERCISE NOTES
_____ minutes

DAILY WRAP-UP
Goals: Exceeded ____ Met ____ Keep Trying ____
Notes:

Success Of The Day:

BY THE NUMBERS: 95: Percent of female college students who didn't meet recommendations for fiber despite being enrolled in a nutrition course, according to one study. **77:** Percent of college women short on iron. **33:** Percent short on calcium.

THURSDAY

SUPPLEMENTS ☐ ☐ WEIGHT ☐

Today's Goals:

MEAL	FOODS & BEVERAGES	FOCUS 1:	FOCUS 2:
BREAKFAST ____ A.M./P.M.			
Hunger:			
Fullness:			
	MEAL TOTALS		
SNACK ____ A.M./P.M.			
Hunger:			
Fullness:			
	MEAL TOTALS		
LUNCH ____ A.M./P.M.			
Hunger:			
Fullness:			
	MEAL TOTALS		
SNACK ____ A.M./P.M.			
Hunger:			
Fullness:			
	MEAL TOTALS		
DINNER ____ A.M./P.M.			
Hunger:			
Fullness:			
	MEAL TOTALS		
	DAILY TOTALS		

EXERCISE NOTES
_____ minutes

DAILY WRAP-UP
Goals: Exceeded ___ Met ___ Keep Trying ___
Notes:

Success Of The Day:

FOOD FACTOID: Working women spend, on average, less than one hour a day preparing, serving, and cleaning up after meals — that's for all meals on a given day. As household income increases, the amount of time women spend preparing food at home decreases.

FRIDAY

SUPPLEMENTS ☐ ☐   WEIGHT ☐

Today's Goals:

MEAL	FOODS & BEVERAGES	FOCUS I:	FOCUS 2:
BREAKFAST ___ A.M./P.M.			
Hunger:			
Fullness:	MEAL TOTALS		
SNACK ___ A.M./P.M.			
Hunger:			
Fullness:	MEAL TOTALS		
LUNCH ___ A.M./P.M.			
Hunger:			
Fullness:	MEAL TOTALS		
SNACK ___ A.M./P.M.			
Hunger:			
Fullness:	MEAL TOTALS		
DINNER ___ A.M./P.M.			
Hunger:			
Fullness:	MEAL TOTALS		
	DAILY TOTALS		

EXERCISE NOTES
_____ minutes

DAILY WRAP-UP
Goals: Exceeded ___ Met ___ Keep Trying ___
Notes:

Success Of The Day:

NUTRITION TIP: If you worry about overeating at parties, bring your own "safety dish" to share, like a veggie platter with salsa, hummus, or bean dip. Keeping your plate full of veggies can help you avoid grabbing a second mini-quiche or fried wonton.

SATURDAY

SUPPLEMENTS ☐ ☐   WEIGHT ☐

Today's Goals:

MEAL	FOODS & BEVERAGES	FOCUS I:	FOCUS 2:
BREAKFAST ___ A.M./P.M.			
Hunger:			
Fullness:			
	MEAL TOTALS		
SNACK ___ A.M./P.M.			
Hunger:			
Fullness:			
	MEAL TOTALS		
LUNCH ___ A.M./P.M.			
Hunger:			
Fullness:			
	MEAL TOTALS		
SNACK ___ A.M./P.M.			
Hunger:			
Fullness:			
	MEAL TOTALS		
DINNER ___ A.M./P.M.			
Hunger:			
Fullness:			
	MEAL TOTALS		
	DAILY TOTALS		

EXERCISE NOTES
_____ minutes

DAILY WRAP-UP
Goals: Exceeded ___ Met ___ Keep Trying ___
Notes:

Success Of The Day:

FITNESS FACTOID: It's important to replace your athletic shoes at least every 6 months if you wear them 3 times a week or more. The shoes should be comfy from the get-go; you shouldn't have to "break them in."

SUNDAY

SUPPLEMENTS ☐ ☐   WEIGHT ☐

Today's Goals:

MEAL	FOODS & BEVERAGES	FOCUS 1:	FOCUS 2:
BREAKFAST ____ A.M./P.M.			
Hunger:			
Fullness:	MEAL TOTALS		
SNACK ____ A.M./P.M.			
Hunger:			
Fullness:	MEAL TOTALS		
LUNCH ____ A.M./P.M.			
Hunger:			
Fullness:	MEAL TOTALS		
SNACK ____ A.M./P.M.			
Hunger:			
Fullness:	MEAL TOTALS		
DINNER ____ A.M./P.M.			
Hunger:			
Fullness:	MEAL TOTALS		
	DAILY TOTALS		

EXERCISE NOTES
_____ minutes

DAILY WRAP-UP
Goals: Exceeded ____ Met ____ Keep Trying ____
Notes:

Success Of The Day:

"If it weren't for the fact that the TV set and the refrigerator are so far apart, some of us wouldn't get any exercise at all." — JOEY ADAMS, comedian

WEEKLY WRAP-UP

SUCCESS OF THE WEEK

GOALS ASSESSMENT

EXERCISE NOTES   **TOTAL DAYS EXERCISED** [ ]   **TOTAL MINUTES/ HOURS** [ ]

PROGRESS REPORT

WHAT WENT WELL, AND WHY?

WHAT DIDN'T GO WELL? WHAT GOT IN MY WAY?

WHAT IS THE MOST IMPORTANT INSIGHT I GAINED ABOUT MYSELF THIS WEEK?

WHAT DO I PLAN TO DO DIFFERENTLY NEXT WEEK?

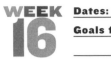

WEEK 16

Dates: _____

Goals for the Week: _____

_____

MONDAY

SUPPLEMENTS ☐ ☐   WEIGHT ☐

Today's Goals: _____

MEAL	FOODS & BEVERAGES	FOCUS I:	FOCUS 2:
BREAKFAST ____ A.M./P.M.			
Hunger:			
Fullness:			
	MEAL TOTALS		
SNACK ____ A.M./P.M.			
Hunger:			
Fullness:			
	MEAL TOTALS		
LUNCH ____ A.M./P.M.			
Hunger:			
Fullness:			
	MEAL TOTALS		
SNACK ____ A.M./P.M.			
Hunger:			
Fullness:			
	MEAL TOTALS		
DINNER ____ A.M./P.M.			
Hunger:			
Fullness:			
	MEAL TOTALS		
	DAILY TOTALS		

EXERCISE NOTES
_____ minutes

DAILY WRAP-UP
Goals: Exceeded ___ Met ___ Keep Trying ___
Notes:

Success Of The Day:

RESEARCH REPORT: Healthy women who skipped breakfast for two weeks ate 100 more calories per day, developed high "bad" (LDL) cholesterol levels, and were less sensitive to insulin than women who ate breakfast daily.

TUESDAY

SUPPLEMENTS ☐ ☐ WEIGHT ☐

Today's Goals: _____

MEAL	FOODS & BEVERAGES	FOCUS I:	FOCUS 2:
BREAKFAST ____ A.M./P.M.			
Hunger:			
Fullness:			
	MEAL TOTALS		
SNACK ____ A.M./P.M.			
Hunger:			
Fullness:			
	MEAL TOTALS		
LUNCH ____ A.M./P.M.			
Hunger:			
Fullness:			
	MEAL TOTALS		
SNACK ____ A.M./P.M.			
Hunger:			
Fullness:			
	MEAL TOTALS		
DINNER ____ A.M./P.M.			
Hunger:			
Fullness:			
	MEAL TOTALS		
	DAILY TOTALS		

EXERCISE NOTES
_____ minutes

DAILY WRAP-UP
Goals: Exceeded ___ Met ___ Keep Trying ___
Notes:

Success Of The Day:

FOOD FACTOID: Americans spend 43 percent of their food dollars on food away from home, a figure expected to rise over the next 20 years by about 18 percent at full-service restaurants and 6 percent for fast food.

FRIDAY

SUPPLEMENTS ☐ ☐   WEIGHT ☐

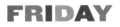

Today's Goals:

MEAL	FOODS & BEVERAGES	FOCUS 1:	FOCUS 2:
BREAKFAST ____ A.M./P.M. Hunger: Fullness:			
	MEAL TOTALS		
SNACK ____ A.M./P.M. Hunger: Fullness:			
	MEAL TOTALS		
LUNCH ____ A.M./P.M. Hunger: Fullness:			
	MEAL TOTALS		
SNACK ____ A.M./P.M. Hunger: Fullness:			
	MEAL TOTALS		
DINNER ____ A.M./P.M. Hunger: Fullness:			
	MEAL TOTALS		
	DAILY TOTALS		

EXERCISE NOTES
_____ minutes

DAILY WRAP-UP
Goals: Exceeded ___ Met ___ Keep Trying ___
Notes:

Success Of The Day:

NUTRITION TIP: Shop the perimeter of the supermarket, where the healthier foods are, and spend little time in the center aisles, home to the processed foods.

SATURDAY

SUPPLEMENTS ☐ ☐   WEIGHT ☐

Today's Goals:

MEAL	FOODS & BEVERAGES	FOCUS I:	FOCUS 2:
BREAKFAST ___ A.M./P.M.			
Hunger:			
Fullness:			
	MEAL TOTALS		
SNACK ___ A.M./P.M.			
Hunger:			
Fullness:			
	MEAL TOTALS		
LUNCH ___ A.M./P.M.			
Hunger:			
Fullness:			
	MEAL TOTALS		
SNACK ___ A.M./P.M.			
Hunger:			
Fullness:			
	MEAL TOTALS		
DINNER ___ A.M./P.M.			
Hunger:			
Fullness:			
	MEAL TOTALS		
	DAILY TOTALS		

EXERCISE NOTES
_____ minutes

DAILY WRAP-UP
Goals: Exceeded ___ Met ___ Keep Trying ___
Notes:

Success Of The Day:

FITNESS FACTOID: In a one-month study, participants who did 90 minutes of Iyengar yoga 3 times a week reported using less pain medication and feeling less anxiety than at the start of the study.

SUNDAY

SUPPLEMENTS ☐ ☐   WEIGHT ☐

Today's Goals: _____

MEAL	FOODS & BEVERAGES	FOCUS I:	FOCUS 2:
BREAKFAST ___ A.M./P.M.			
Hunger:			
Fullness:			
	MEAL TOTALS		
SNACK ___ A.M./P.M.			
Hunger:			
Fullness:			
	MEAL TOTALS		
LUNCH ___ A.M./P.M.			
Hunger:			
Fullness:			
	MEAL TOTALS		
SNACK ___ A.M./P.M.			
Hunger:			
Fullness:			
	MEAL TOTALS		
DINNER ___ A.M./P.M.			
Hunger:			
Fullness:			
	MEAL TOTALS		
	DAILY TOTALS		

EXERCISE NOTES
_____ minutes

DAILY WRAP-UP
Goals: Exceeded ___ Met ___ Keep Trying ___
Notes:

Success Of The Day:

"Dinner is and always was a great artistic opportunity."

WEEKLY WRAP-UP

SUCCESS OF THE WEEK

GOALS ASSESSMENT

EXERCISE NOTES	**TOTAL DAYS EXERCISED**		**TOTAL MINUTES/ HOURS**	

PROGRESS REPORT

WHAT WENT WELL, AND WHY?

WHAT DIDN'T GO WELL? WHAT GOT IN MY WAY?

WHAT IS THE MOST IMPORTANT INSIGHT I GAINED ABOUT MYSELF THIS WEEK?

WHAT DO I PLAN TO DO DIFFERENTLY NEXT WEEK?

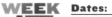

WEEK 17

Dates: _____

Goals for the Week: _____

_____

MONDAY

SUPPLEMENTS [____] [____]   WEIGHT [____]

Today's Goals: _____

MEAL	FOODS & BEVERAGES	FOCUS I:	FOCUS 2:
BREAKFAST ____ A.M./P.M.			
Hunger:			
Fullness:			
	MEAL TOTALS		
SNACK ____ A.M./P.M.			
Hunger:			
Fullness:			
	MEAL TOTALS		
LUNCH ____ A.M./P.M.			
Hunger:			
Fullness:			
	MEAL TOTALS		
SNACK ____ A.M./P.M.			
Hunger:			
Fullness:			
	MEAL TOTALS		
DINNER ____ A.M./P.M.			
Hunger:			
Fullness:			
	MEAL TOTALS		
	DAILY TOTALS		

EXERCISE NOTES
_____ minutes

DAILY WRAP-UP
Goals: Exceeded ____ Met ____ Keep Trying ____
Notes:
Success Of The Day:

RESEARCH REPORT: Even when food doesn't taste good, people eat more out of a large container than a small one. In one study, moviegoers who were offered stale popcorn ate 61 percent more when given a large container than a small one.

TUESDAY

SUPPLEMENTS ☐ ☐   WEIGHT ☐

Today's Goals:

MEAL	FOODS & BEVERAGES	FOCUS 1:	FOCUS 2:
BREAKFAST ___ A.M./P.M.			
Hunger:			
Fullness:			
	MEAL TOTALS		
SNACK ___ A.M./P.M.			
Hunger:			
Fullness:			
	MEAL TOTALS		
LUNCH ___ A.M./P.M.			
Hunger:			
Fullness:			
	MEAL TOTALS		
SNACK ___ A.M./P.M.			
Hunger:			
Fullness:			
	MEAL TOTALS		
DINNER ___ A.M./P.M.			
Hunger:			
Fullness:			
	MEAL TOTALS		
	DAILY TOTALS		

EXERCISE NOTES
_____ minutes

DAILY WRAP-UP
Goals: Exceeded ___ Met ___ Keep Trying ___
Notes:

Success Of The Day:

NUTRITION SHOCKER: A croissant in France weighs about 2 ounces and contains 215 calories. In the United States, a croissant typically weighs 4 ounces and contains 430 calories.

WEDNESDAY

SUPPLEMENTS ☐ ☐ WEIGHT ☐

Today's Goals: _____

MEAL	FOODS & BEVERAGES	FOCUS I:	FOCUS 2:
BREAKFAST ___ A.M./P.M.			
Hunger:			
Fullness:			
	MEAL TOTALS		
SNACK ___ A.M./P.M.			
Hunger:			
Fullness:			
	MEAL TOTALS		
LUNCH ___ A.M./P.M.			
Hunger:			
Fullness:			
	MEAL TOTALS		
SNACK ___ A.M./P.M.			
Hunger:			
Fullness:			
	MEAL TOTALS		
DINNER ___ A.M./P.M.			
Hunger:			
Fullness:			
	MEAL TOTALS		
	DAILY TOTALS		

EXERCISE NOTES
_____ minutes

DAILY WRAP-UP
Goals: Exceeded ___ Met ___ Keep Trying ___
Notes:

Success Of The Day:

BY THE NUMBERS: 91,000: Number of calories you'll save in a year if you give up one daily 20-ounce soda. **7,280:** Number of teaspoons of sugar you'll skip. **26:** Number of pounds you could potentially lose, all else being equal.

THURSDAY

SUPPLEMENTS ☐ ☐ WEIGHT ☐

Today's Goals:

MEAL	FOODS & BEVERAGES	FOCUS 1:	FOCUS 2:
BREAKFAST ___ A.M./P.M.			
Hunger:			
Fullness:			
	MEAL TOTALS		
SNACK ___ A.M./P.M.			
Hunger:			
Fullness:			
	MEAL TOTALS		
LUNCH ___ A.M./P.M.			
Hunger:			
Fullness:			
	MEAL TOTALS		
SNACK ___ A.M./P.M.			
Hunger:			
Fullness:			
	MEAL TOTALS		
DINNER ___ A.M./P.M.			
Hunger:			
Fullness:			
	MEAL TOTALS		
	DAILY TOTALS		

EXERCISE NOTES
_____ minutes

DAILY WRAP-UP
Goals: Exceeded ___ Met ___ Keep Trying ___
Notes:

Success Of The Day:

FOOD FACTOID: When children get a voice in the family's meal planning and help out in the kitchen, they have more buy-in and are more likely to become adventurous eaters. Let your little ones stir ingredients, wash lettuce, and help pack lunches.

FRIDAY

SUPPLEMENTS ☐ ☐   WEIGHT ☐

Today's Goals:

MEAL	FOODS & BEVERAGES	FOCUS I:	FOCUS 2:
BREAKFAST ___ A.M./P.M.			
Hunger:			
Fullness:			
	MEAL TOTALS		
SNACK ___ A.M./P.M.			
Hunger:			
Fullness:			
	MEAL TOTALS		
LUNCH ___ A.M./P.M.			
Hunger:			
Fullness:			
	MEAL TOTALS		
SNACK ___ A.M./P.M.			
Hunger:			
Fullness:			
	MEAL TOTALS		
DINNER ___ A.M./P.M.			
Hunger:			
Fullness:			
	MEAL TOTALS		
	DAILY TOTALS		

EXERCISE NOTES
_____ minutes

DAILY WRAP-UP
Goals: Exceeded ___ Met ___ Keep Trying ___
Notes:

Success Of The Day:

NUTRITION TIP: If, like many Americans, you grill often, remember that one portion of meat is 3 ounces cooked, about the thickness and width of a deck of cards. That means I pound (16 ounces) of raw chicken breast should serve about four people.

SATURDAY

SUPPLEMENTS ☐ ☐   WEIGHT ☐

Today's Goals:

MEAL	FOODS & BEVERAGES	FOCUS 1:	FOCUS 2:
BREAKFAST ___ A.M./P.M. Hunger: Fullness:			
	MEAL TOTALS		
SNACK ___ A.M./P.M. Hunger: Fullness:			
	MEAL TOTALS		
LUNCH ___ A.M./P.M. Hunger: Fullness:			
	MEAL TOTALS		
SNACK ___ A.M./P.M. Hunger: Fullness:			
	MEAL TOTALS		
DINNER ___ A.M./P.M. Hunger: Fullness:			
	MEAL TOTALS		
	DAILY TOTALS		

EXERCISE NOTES
_____ minutes

DAILY WRAP-UP
Goals: Exceeded ___ Met ___ Keep Trying ___
Notes:

Success Of The Day:

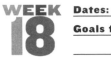

Dates: _____

Goals for the Week: _____

_____

MONDAY

SUPPLEMENTS ☐ ☐ WEIGHT ☐

Today's Goals:

MEAL	FOODS & BEVERAGES	FOCUS I:	FOCUS 2:
BREAKFAST ___ A.M./P.M.			
Hunger:			
Fullness:			
	MEAL TOTALS		
SNACK ___ A.M./P.M.			
Hunger:			
Fullness:			
	MEAL TOTALS		
LUNCH ___ A.M./P.M.			
Hunger:			
Fullness:			
	MEAL TOTALS		
SNACK ___ A.M./P.M.			
Hunger:			
Fullness:			
	MEAL TOTALS		
DINNER ___ A.M./P.M.			
Hunger:			
Fullness:			
	MEAL TOTALS		
	DAILY TOTALS		

EXERCISE NOTES
_____ minutes

DAILY WRAP-UP

Goals: Exceeded ___ Met ___ Keep Trying ___

Notes:

Success Of The Day:

RESEARCH REPORT: Drinking water doesn't help you feel full, but eating foods high in water, such as soups and produce, does help. Women ate 100 fewer calories when served a chicken-and-rice soup than when served a casserole with the same ingredients and calorie count, plus a glass of water.

TUESDAY

SUPPLEMENTS ☐ ☐   WEIGHT ☐

Today's Goals: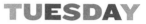

MEAL	FOODS & BEVERAGES	FOCUS 1:	FOCUS 2:
BREAKFAST ____ A.M./P.M. Hunger: Fullness:			
	MEAL TOTALS		
SNACK ____ A.M./P.M. Hunger: Fullness:			
	MEAL TOTALS		
LUNCH ____ A.M./P.M. Hunger: Fullness:			
	MEAL TOTALS		
SNACK ____ A.M./P.M. Hunger: Fullness:			
	MEAL TOTALS		
DINNER ____ A.M./P.M. Hunger: Fullness:			
	MEAL TOTALS		
	DAILY TOTALS		

EXERCISE NOTES
_____ minutes

DAILY WRAP-UP
Goals: Exceeded ___ Met ___ Keep Trying ___
Notes:

Success Of The Day:

FOOD FACTOID: Yogurt and soy milk products that boast about containing omega-3 fatty acids typically contain only tiny amounts of **DHA**, the type of omega-3 fat that is linked to heart and brain health. Many contain the same amount of **DHA** that's in a bite of salmon.

FRIDAY

SUPPLEMENTS ☐ ☐ WEIGHT ☐

Today's Goals:

MEAL	FOODS & BEVERAGES	FOCUS I:	FOCUS 2:
BREAKFAST ___ A.M./P.M.			
Hunger:			
Fullness:			
	MEAL TOTALS		
SNACK ___ A.M./P.M.			
Hunger:			
Fullness:			
	MEAL TOTALS		
LUNCH ___ A.M./P.M.			
Hunger:			
Fullness:			
	MEAL TOTALS		
SNACK ___ A.M./P.M.			
Hunger:			
Fullness:			
	MEAL TOTALS		
DINNER ___ A.M./P.M.			
Hunger:			
Fullness:			
	MEAL TOTALS		
	DAILY TOTALS		

EXERCISE NOTES
_____ minutes

DAILY WRAP-UP
Goals: Exceeded ___ Met ___ Keep Trying ___
Notes:

Success Of The Day:

NUTRITION TIP: Instead of topping frozen whole-grain waffles with syrup, use warmed-up frozen fruit such as berries, cherries, or peaches. One cup of frozen fruit provides about 100 fewer calories than ¼ cup of maple syrup.

SATURDAY

SUPPLEMENTS ☐ ☐   WEIGHT ☐

Today's Goals:

MEAL	FOODS & BEVERAGES	FOCUS I:	FOCUS 2:
BREAKFAST ___ A.M./P.M.			
Hunger:			
Fullness:			
	MEAL TOTALS		
SNACK ___ A.M./P.M.			
Hunger:			
Fullness:			
	MEAL TOTALS		
LUNCH ___ A.M./P.M.			
Hunger:			
Fullness:			
	MEAL TOTALS		
SNACK ___ A.M./P.M.			
Hunger:			
Fullness:			
	MEAL TOTALS		
DINNER ___ A.M./P.M.			
Hunger:			
Fullness:			
	MEAL TOTALS		
	DAILY TOTALS		

EXERCISE NOTES
_____ minutes

DAILY WRAP-UP
Goals: Exceeded ___ Met ___ Keep Trying ___
Notes:

Success Of The Day:

FITNESS FACTOID: A huge body of research shows that exercise — at least 30 minutes 3 to 5 days a week — can help improve symptoms of depression and anxiety and prevent a relapse after treatment for these conditions.

SUNDAY

SUPPLEMENTS ☐ ☐   WEIGHT ☐

Today's Goals:

MEAL	FOODS & BEVERAGES	FOCUS I:	FOCUS 2:
BREAKFAST ___ A.M./P.M.			
Hunger:			
Fullness:			
	MEAL TOTALS		
SNACK ___ A.M./P.M.			
Hunger:			
Fullness:			
	MEAL TOTALS		
LUNCH ___ A.M./P.M.			
Hunger:			
Fullness:			
	MEAL TOTALS		
SNACK ___ A.M./P.M.			
Hunger:			
Fullness:			
	MEAL TOTALS		
DINNER ___ A.M./P.M.			
Hunger:			
Fullness:			
	MEAL TOTALS		
	DAILY TOTALS		

EXERCISE NOTES
_____ minutes

DAILY WRAP-UP
Goals: Exceeded ___   Met ___   Keep Trying ___
Notes:

Success Of The Day:

"If hunger is not the problem, then eating is not the solution."

WEEKLY WRAP-UP

SUCCESS OF THE WEEK

GOALS ASSESSMENT

EXERCISE NOTES	**TOTAL DAYS EXERCISED**	**TOTAL MINUTES/ HOURS**

PROGRESS REPORT

WHAT WENT WELL, AND WHY?

WHAT DIDN'T GO WELL? WHAT GOT IN MY WAY?

WHAT IS THE MOST IMPORTANT INSIGHT I GAINED ABOUT MYSELF THIS WEEK?

WHAT DO I PLAN TO DO DIFFERENTLY NEXT WEEK?

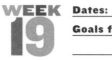

WEEK 19

Dates: _____

Goals for the Week: _____

_____

MONDAY

SUPPLEMENTS ☐ ☐   WEIGHT ☐

Today's Goals: _____

MEAL	FOODS & BEVERAGES	FOCUS 1:	FOCUS 2:
BREAKFAST ____ A.M./P.M.			
Hunger:			
Fullness:	MEAL TOTALS		
SNACK ____ A.M./P.M.			
Hunger:			
Fullness:	MEAL TOTALS		
LUNCH ____ A.M./P.M.			
Hunger:			
Fullness:	MEAL TOTALS		
SNACK ____ A.M./P.M.			
Hunger:			
Fullness:	MEAL TOTALS		
DINNER ____ A.M./P.M.			
Hunger:			
Fullness:	MEAL TOTALS		
	DAILY TOTALS		

EXERCISE NOTES
_____ minutes

DAILY WRAP-UP
Goals: Exceeded ___ Met ___ Keep Trying ___
Notes:

Success Of The Day:

RESEARCH REPORT: In one study, women who added 2 ounces of almonds (about 344 calories' worth) to their diets for 10 weeks didn't gain weight. They naturally ate fewer calories throughout the day, probably because the protein, fat, and fiber in the almonds kept them satisfied.

TUESDAY

SUPPLEMENTS ☐ ☐   WEIGHT ☐

Today's Goals:

MEAL	FOODS & BEVERAGES	FOCUS 1:	FOCUS 2:
BREAKFAST ____ A.M./P.M.			
Hunger:			
Fullness:			
	MEAL TOTALS		
SNACK ____ A.M./P.M.			
Hunger:			
Fullness:			
	MEAL TOTALS		
LUNCH ____ A.M./P.M.			
Hunger:			
Fullness:			
	MEAL TOTALS		
SNACK ____ A.M./P.M.			
Hunger:			
Fullness:			
	MEAL TOTALS		
DINNER ____ A.M./P.M.			
Hunger:			
Fullness:			
	MEAL TOTALS		
	DAILY TOTALS		

EXERCISE NOTES
_____ minutes

DAILY WRAP-UP
Goals: Exceeded ____ Met ____ Keep Trying ____
Notes:

Success Of The Day:

NUTRITION SHOCKER: Soft drinks comprise as much as 15 percent of the calorie intake of teenage girls in the United States. Soda is the number one beverage choice of teenage girls.

WEDNESDAY SUPPLEMENTS ☐ ☐ WEIGHT ☐

Today's Goals:

MEAL	FOODS & BEVERAGES	FOCUS I:	FOCUS 2:
BREAKFAST ____ A.M./P.M.			
Hunger:			
Fullness:			
	MEAL TOTALS		
SNACK ____ A.M./P.M.			
Hunger:			
Fullness:			
	MEAL TOTALS		
LUNCH ____ A.M./P.M.			
Hunger:			
Fullness:			
	MEAL TOTALS		
SNACK ____ A.M./P.M.			
Hunger:			
Fullness:			
	MEAL TOTALS		
DINNER ____ A.M./P.M.			
Hunger:			
Fullness:			
	MEAL TOTALS		
	DAILY TOTALS		

EXERCISE NOTES
_____ minutes

DAILY WRAP-UP
Goals: Exceeded ____ Met ____ Keep Trying ____
Notes:

Success Of The Day:

BY THE NUMBERS: 44: Number of ingredients in Kellogg's Chocolate Pop-Tarts, most of which are preservatives, artificial colors and flavors, and added sugars. **39:** Number of ingredients in a Twinkie. **1:** Number of ingredients in Quick Quaker Oats.

THURSDAY

SUPPLEMENTS ☐ ☐   WEIGHT ☐

Today's Goals: _____

MEAL	FOODS & BEVERAGES	FOCUS 1:	FOCUS 2:
BREAKFAST ___ A.M./P.M.			
Hunger:			
Fullness:			
	MEAL TOTALS		
SNACK ___ A.M./P.M.			
Hunger:			
Fullness:			
	MEAL TOTALS		
LUNCH ___ A.M./P.M.			
Hunger:			
Fullness:			
	MEAL TOTALS		
SNACK ___ A.M./P.M.			
Hunger:			
Fullness:			
	MEAL TOTALS		
DINNER ___ A.M./P.M.			
Hunger:			
Fullness:			
	MEAL TOTALS		
	DAILY TOTALS		

EXERCISE NOTES
_____ minutes

DAILY WRAP-UP
Goals: Exceeded ___ Met ___ Keep Trying ___
Notes:

Success Of The Day:

FOOD FACTOID: On a typical day, more than 40 percent of Americans eat at a restaurant.

FRIDAY

SUPPLEMENTS ☐☐ WEIGHT ☐

Today's Goals:

MEAL	FOODS & BEVERAGES	FOCUS I:	FOCUS 2:
BREAKFAST ___ A.M./P.M.			
Hunger:			
Fullness:			
	MEAL TOTALS		
SNACK ___ A.M./P.M.			
Hunger:			
Fullness:			
	MEAL TOTALS		
LUNCH ___ A.M./P.M.			
Hunger:			
Fullness:			
	MEAL TOTALS		
SNACK ___ A.M./P.M.			
Hunger:			
Fullness:			
	MEAL TOTALS		
DINNER ___ A.M./P.M.			
Hunger:			
Fullness:			
	MEAL TOTALS		
	DAILY TOTALS		

EXERCISE NOTES
_____ minutes

DAILY WRAP-UP
Goals: Exceeded ___ Met ___ Keep Trying ___
Notes:

Success Of The Day:

NUTRITION TIP: The average worker takes 31 minutes for lunch, down from 36 minutes in 1996. If you have a half hour, carve out 5 to 10 minutes for a brisk walk, and bring a balanced meal, like greens with canned salmon, low-fat cheese, nuts, whole-wheat crackers, and a pear.

SATURDAY

SUPPLEMENTS ☐ ☐ WEIGHT ☐

Today's Goals:

MEAL	FOODS & BEVERAGES	FOCUS 1:	FOCUS 2:
BREAKFAST ___ A.M./P.M.			
Hunger:			
Fullness:			
	MEAL TOTALS		
SNACK ___ A.M./P.M.			
Hunger:			
Fullness:			
	MEAL TOTALS		
LUNCH ___ A.M./P.M.			
Hunger:			
Fullness:			
	MEAL TOTALS		
SNACK ___ A.M./P.M.			
Hunger:			
Fullness:			
	MEAL TOTALS		
DINNER ___ A.M./P.M.			
Hunger:			
Fullness:			
	MEAL TOTALS		
	DAILY TOTALS		

EXERCISE NOTES
_____ minutes

DAILY WRAP-UP
Goals: Exceeded ___ Met ___ Keep Trying ___
Notes:

Success Of The Day:

FITNESS FACTOID: Multiple short bouts of exercise can be just as effective for fitness and weight loss as one long workout. In one study, subjects who exercised for three 10-minute sessions a day reaped the same benefits as subjects who did one 30-minute session.

SUNDAY

SUPPLEMENTS [   ] [   ]   WEIGHT [   ]

Today's Goals:

MEAL	FOODS & BEVERAGES	FOCUS 1:	FOCUS 2:
BREAKFAST ___ A.M./P.M.			
Hunger:			
Fullness:			
	MEAL TOTALS		
SNACK ___ A.M./P.M.			
Hunger:			
Fullness:			
	MEAL TOTALS		
LUNCH ___ A.M./P.M.			
Hunger:			
Fullness:			
	MEAL TOTALS		
SNACK ___ A.M./P.M.			
Hunger:			
Fullness:			
	MEAL TOTALS		
DINNER ___ A.M./P.M.			
Hunger:			
Fullness:			
	MEAL TOTALS		
	DAILY TOTALS		

EXERCISE NOTES
_____ minutes

DAILY WRAP-UP
Goals: Exceeded ___ Met ___ Keep Trying ___
Notes:

Success Of The Day:

"Nothing will benefit human health and increase the chances for survival of life on Earth as much as the evolution to a vegetarian diet."

— ALBERT EINSTEIN

WEEKLY WRAP-UP

SUCCESS OF THE WEEK

GOALS ASSESSMENT

EXERCISE NOTES   **TOTAL DAYS EXERCISED** [ ]   **TOTAL MINUTES/ HOURS** [ ]

PROGRESS REPORT

WHAT WENT WELL, AND WHY?

WHAT DIDN'T GO WELL? WHAT GOT IN MY WAY?

WHAT IS THE MOST IMPORTANT INSIGHT I GAINED ABOUT MYSELF THIS WEEK?

WHAT DO I PLAN TO DO DIFFERENTLY NEXT WEEK?

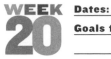

WEEK
20

Dates: _____

Goals for the Week: _____
_____

MONDAY

SUPPLEMENTS ☐ ☐ WEIGHT ☐

Today's Goals: _____

MEAL	FOODS & BEVERAGES	FOCUS 1:	FOCUS 2:
BREAKFAST ___ A.M./P.M.			
Hunger:			
Fullness:			
	MEAL TOTALS		
SNACK ___ A.M./P.M.			
Hunger:			
Fullness:			
	MEAL TOTALS		
LUNCH ___ A.M./P.M.			
Hunger:			
Fullness:			
	MEAL TOTALS		
SNACK ___ A.M./P.M.			
Hunger:			
Fullness:			
	MEAL TOTALS		
DINNER ___ A.M./P.M.			
Hunger:			
Fullness:			
	MEAL TOTALS		
	DAILY TOTALS		

EXERCISE NOTES
_____ minutes

DAILY WRAP-UP
Goals: Exceeded ___ Met ___ Keep Trying ___
Notes:

Success Of The Day:

RESEARCH REPORT: Studies show that compared to a typical Western diet — high in processed foods, refined sugars, and cured and red meats — a Mediterranean diet reduces the risk of lung diseases such as emphysema and bronchitis by 50 percent.

TUESDAY

SUPPLEMENTS ☐ ☐ WEIGHT ☐

Today's Goals:

MEAL	FOODS & BEVERAGES	FOCUS I:	FOCUS 2:
BREAKFAST ___ A.M./P.M.			
Hunger:			
Fullness:	MEAL TOTALS		
SNACK ___ A.M./P.M.			
Hunger:			
Fullness:	MEAL TOTALS		
LUNCH ___ A.M./P.M.			
Hunger:			
Fullness:	MEAL TOTALS		
SNACK ___ A.M./P.M.			
Hunger:			
Fullness:	MEAL TOTALS		
DINNER ___ A.M./P.M.			
Hunger:			
Fullness:	MEAL TOTALS		
	DAILY TOTALS		

EXERCISE NOTES
_____ minutes

DAILY WRAP-UP
Goals: Exceeded ___ Met ___ Keep Trying ___
Notes:

Success Of The Day:

NUTRITION SHOCKER: Of America's 15 top-rated hospitals, 6 have fast-food franchises in the lobby.

WEDNESDAY

SUPPLEMENTS ☐ ☐   WEIGHT ☐

Today's Goals:

MEAL	FOODS & BEVERAGES	FOCUS I:	FOCUS 2:
BREAKFAST ____ A.M./P.M.			
Hunger:			
Fullness:	MEAL TOTALS		
SNACK ____ A.M./P.M.			
Hunger:			
Fullness:	MEAL TOTALS		
LUNCH ____ A.M./P.M.			
Hunger:			
Fullness:	MEAL TOTALS		
SNACK ____ A.M./P.M.			
Hunger:			
Fullness:	MEAL TOTALS		
DINNER ____ A.M./P.M.			
Hunger:			
Fullness:	MEAL TOTALS		
	DAILY TOTALS		

EXERCISE NOTES
_____ minutes

DAILY WRAP-UP
Goals: Exceeded ____ Met ____ Keep Trying ____
Notes:

Success Of The Day:

BY THE NUMBERS: 2,300: Maximum number, in milligrams, of daily sodium intake recommended by the latest dietary guidelines. **3,011:** The average milligrams of sodium consumed daily by women 31 to 50 years old. **4,252:** Average milligrams of sodium consumed daily by men.

THURSDAY

SUPPLEMENTS ☐ ☐ WEIGHT ☐

Today's Goals:

MEAL	FOODS & BEVERAGES	FOCUS 1:	FOCUS 2:
BREAKFAST ___ A.M./P.M.			
Hunger:			
Fullness:			
	MEAL TOTALS		
SNACK ___ A.M./P.M.			
Hunger:			
Fullness:			
	MEAL TOTALS		
LUNCH ___ A.M./P.M.			
Hunger:			
Fullness:			
	MEAL TOTALS		
SNACK ___ A.M./P.M.			
Hunger:			
Fullness:			
	MEAL TOTALS		
DINNER ___ A.M./P.M.			
Hunger:			
Fullness:			
	MEAL TOTALS		
	DAILY TOTALS		

EXERCISE NOTES
_____ minutes

DAILY WRAP-UP
Goals: Exceeded ___ Met ___ Keep Trying ___
Notes:

Success Of The Day:

FOOD FACTOID: About 20 percent of the total calories in a typical American diet are from added sugars, including sweetened drinks, candy, and baked goods. The largest source is soft drinks, followed by table sugar.

FRIDAY

SUPPLEMENTS ☐ ☐   WEIGHT ☐

Today's Goals:

MEAL	FOODS & BEVERAGES	FOCUS 1:	FOCUS 2:
BREAKFAST ___ A.M./P.M.			
Hunger:			
Fullness:			
	MEAL TOTALS		
SNACK ___ A.M./P.M.			
Hunger:			
Fullness:			
	MEAL TOTALS		
LUNCH ___ A.M./P.M.			
Hunger:			
Fullness:			
	MEAL TOTALS		
SNACK ___ A.M./P.M.			
Hunger:			
Fullness:			
	MEAL TOTALS		
DINNER ___ A.M./P.M.			
Hunger:			
Fullness:			
	MEAL TOTALS		
	DAILY TOTALS		

EXERCISE NOTES
___ minutes

DAILY WRAP-UP
Goals: Exceeded ___   Met ___   Keep Trying ___
Notes:

Success Of The Day:

NUTRITION TIP: If you rely on energy bars as meal replacements, choose a bar with 15 grams of carbohydrate (same as 1 slice of bread), 7 grams of protein (same as 1 ounce of lean meat), and 5 grams of fat (same as 1 teaspoon of oil).

SATURDAY

SUPPLEMENTS ☐ ☐   WEIGHT ☐

Today's Goals:

MEAL	FOODS & BEVERAGES	FOCUS 1:	FOCUS 2:
BREAKFAST ___ A.M./P.M.			
Hunger:			
Fullness:			
	MEAL TOTALS		
SNACK ___ A.M./P.M.			
Hunger:			
Fullness:			
	MEAL TOTALS		
LUNCH ___ A.M./P.M.			
Hunger:			
Fullness:			
	MEAL TOTALS		
SNACK ___ A.M./P.M.			
Hunger:			
Fullness:			
	MEAL TOTALS		
DINNER ___ A.M./P.M.			
Hunger:			
Fullness:			
	MEAL TOTALS		
	DAILY TOTALS		

EXERCISE NOTES
_____ minutes

DAILY WRAP-UP
Goals: Exceeded ___ Met ___ Keep Trying ___
Notes:

Success Of The Day:

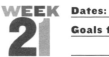

WEEK 21

Dates: _____

Goals for the Week: _____

_____

MONDAY

SUPPLEMENTS ☐ ☐ WEIGHT ☐

Today's Goals: _____

MEAL	FOODS & BEVERAGES	FOCUS 1:	FOCUS 2:
BREAKFAST ___ A.M./P.M.			
Hunger:			
Fullness:	MEAL TOTALS		
SNACK ___ A.M./P.M.			
Hunger:			
Fullness:	MEAL TOTALS		
LUNCH ___ A.M./P.M.			
Hunger:			
Fullness:	MEAL TOTALS		
SNACK ___ A.M./P.M.			
Hunger:			
Fullness:	MEAL TOTALS		
DINNER ___ A.M./P.M.			
Hunger:			
Fullness:	MEAL TOTALS		
	DAILY TOTALS		

EXERCISE NOTES
_____ minutes

DAILY WRAP-UP
Goals: Exceeded ___ Met ___ Keep Trying ___
Notes:

Success Of The Day:

RESEARCH REPORT: You can boost your intake of nutritious foods and drinks by making them more convenient. In a mess-hall study, soldiers drank 42 percent more milk when the milk machine was 12 feet away from the table than when it was 25 feet away.

TUESDAY

SUPPLEMENTS ☐ ☐ WEIGHT ☐

Today's Goals: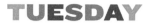

MEAL	FOODS & BEVERAGES	FOCUS 1:	FOCUS 2:
BREAKFAST ___ A.M./P.M.			
Hunger:			
Fullness:			
	MEAL TOTALS		
SNACK ___ A.M./P.M.			
Hunger:			
Fullness:			
	MEAL TOTALS		
LUNCH ___ A.M./P.M.			
Hunger:			
Fullness:			
	MEAL TOTALS		
SNACK ___ A.M./P.M.			
Hunger:			
Fullness:			
	MEAL TOTALS		
DINNER ___ A.M./P.M.			
Hunger:			
Fullness:			
	MEAL TOTALS		
	DAILY TOTALS		

EXERCISE NOTES
_____ minutes

DAILY WRAP-UP
Goals: Exceeded ___ Met ___ Keep Trying ___
Notes:

Success Of The Day:

NUTRITION SHOCKER: When researchers asked Subway patrons to guess the calorie count of a 911-calorie meal they'd just eaten, they guessed 559.

WEDNESDAY   SUPPLEMENTS ☐ ☐   WEIGHT ☐

Today's Goals:

MEAL	FOODS & BEVERAGES	FOCUS 1:	FOCUS 2:
BREAKFAST ____ A.M./P.M.			
Hunger:			
Fullness:			
	MEAL TOTALS		
SNACK ____ A.M./P.M.			
Hunger:			
Fullness:			
	MEAL TOTALS		
LUNCH ____ A.M./P.M.			
Hunger:			
Fullness:			
	MEAL TOTALS		
SNACK ____ A.M./P.M.			
Hunger:			
Fullness:			
	MEAL TOTALS		
DINNER ____ A.M./P.M.			
Hunger:			
Fullness:			
	MEAL TOTALS		
	DAILY TOTALS		

EXERCISE NOTES
_____ minutes

DAILY WRAP-UP
Goals: Exceeded ____ Met ____ Keep Trying ____
Notes:

Success Of The Day:

BY THE NUMBERS: 100: Number, in acres, of pizza eaten every day by Americans. **350:** Number of pizza slices eaten per second. **459:** Calories in one slice of Sbarro's cheese pizza.

THURSDAY

SUPPLEMENTS ☐ ☐   WEIGHT ☐

Today's Goals:

MEAL	FOODS & BEVERAGES	FOCUS I:	FOCUS 2:
BREAKFAST ____ A.M./P.M.			
Hunger:			
Fullness:			
	MEAL TOTALS		
SNACK ____ A.M./P.M.			
Hunger:			
Fullness:			
	MEAL TOTALS		
LUNCH ____ A.M./P.M.			
Hunger:			
Fullness:			
	MEAL TOTALS		
SNACK ____ A.M./P.M.			
Hunger:			
Fullness:			
	MEAL TOTALS		
DINNER ____ A.M./P.M.			
Hunger:			
Fullness:			
	MEAL TOTALS		
	DAILY TOTALS		

EXERCISE NOTES
_____ minutes

DAILY WRAP-UP
Goals: Exceeded ____ Met ____ Keep Trying ____
Notes:

Success Of The Day:

FOOD FACTOID: Seafood is the richest source of omega-3 fats, essential for heart health and infant brain development and possibly valuable for fighting mental decline, depression, stroke, and inflammation. Eating 6 ounces of fatty fish per week reduces coronary death risk by 36 percent.

FRIDAY

SUPPLEMENTS ☐ ☐   WEIGHT ☐

Today's Goals:

MEAL	FOODS & BEVERAGES	FOCUS I:	FOCUS 2:
BREAKFAST ____ A.M./P.M.			
Hunger:			
Fullness:			
	MEAL TOTALS		
SNACK ____ A.M./P.M.			
Hunger:			
Fullness:			
	MEAL TOTALS		
LUNCH ____ A.M./P.M.			
Hunger:			
Fullness:			
	MEAL TOTALS		
SNACK ____ A.M./P.M.			
Hunger:			
Fullness:			
	MEAL TOTALS		
DINNER ____ A.M./P.M.			
Hunger:			
Fullness:			
	MEAL TOTALS		
	DAILY TOTALS		

EXERCISE NOTES
_____ minutes

DAILY WRAP-UP
Goals: Exceeded ____   Met ____   Keep Trying ____
Notes:

Success Of The Day:

NUTRITION TIP: Use spices and extracts to flavor coffee and oatmeal in place of sugar. A drop or two of vanilla extract or a sprinkle of cinnamon, nutmeg, cloves, or even spice blends like pumpkin and apple pie will make your taste buds happy and curb your craving for sweets.

SATURDAY

SUPPLEMENTS ☐ ☐ WEIGHT ☐

Today's Goals:

MEAL	FOODS & BEVERAGES	FOCUS I:	FOCUS 2:
BREAKFAST ___ A.M./P.M. Hunger: Fullness:			
	MEAL TOTALS		
SNACK ___ A.M./P.M. Hunger: Fullness:			
	MEAL TOTALS		
LUNCH ___ A.M./P.M. Hunger: Fullness:			
	MEAL TOTALS		
SNACK ___ A.M./P.M. Hunger: Fullness:			
	MEAL TOTALS		
DINNER ___ A.M./P.M. Hunger: Fullness:			
	MEAL TOTALS		
	DAILY TOTALS		

EXERCISE NOTES
_____ minutes

DAILY WRAP-UP
Goals: Exceeded ___ Met ___ Keep Trying ___
Notes:

Success Of The Day:

FITNESS FACTOID: Substantial research shows that moderate exercise can boost immunity. The average adult gets two to five colds per year. Regular workouts can reduce this number by 25 percent.

SUNDAY

SUPPLEMENTS ☐ ☐ WEIGHT ☐

Today's Goals:

MEAL	FOODS & BEVERAGES	FOCUS I:	FOCUS 2:
BREAKFAST _____ A.M./P.M.			
Hunger:			
Fullness:	MEAL TOTALS		
SNACK _____ A.M./P.M.			
Hunger:			
Fullness:	MEAL TOTALS		
LUNCH _____ A.M./P.M.			
Hunger:			
Fullness:	MEAL TOTALS		
SNACK _____ A.M./P.M.			
Hunger:			
Fullness:	MEAL TOTALS		
DINNER _____ A.M./P.M.			
Hunger:			
Fullness:	MEAL TOTALS		
	DAILY TOTALS		

EXERCISE NOTES
_____ minutes

DAILY WRAP-UP
Goals: Exceeded ___ Met ___ Keep Trying ___
Notes:

Success Of The Day:

"I'm not overweight. I'm just nine inches too short."   — SHELLEY WINTERS

WEEKLY WRAP-UP

SUCCESS OF THE WEEK

GOALS ASSESSMENT

EXERCISE NOTES   **TOTAL DAYS EXERCISED** [ ]   **TOTAL MINUTES/ HOURS** [ ]

PROGRESS REPORT

WHAT WENT WELL, AND WHY?

WHAT DIDN'T GO WELL? WHAT GOT IN MY WAY?

WHAT IS THE MOST IMPORTANT INSIGHT I GAINED ABOUT MYSELF THIS WEEK?

WHAT DO I PLAN TO DO DIFFERENTLY NEXT WEEK?

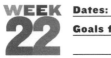
WEEK
22

Dates: _____

Goals for the Week: _____

_____

MONDAY

SUPPLEMENTS ☐ ☐   WEIGHT ☐

Today's Goals: _____

MEAL	FOODS & BEVERAGES	FOCUS I:	FOCUS 2:
BREAKFAST ____ A.M./P.M.			
Hunger:			
Fullness:			
	MEAL TOTALS		
SNACK ____ A.M./P.M.			
Hunger:			
Fullness:			
	MEAL TOTALS		
LUNCH ____ A.M./P.M.			
Hunger:			
Fullness:			
	MEAL TOTALS		
SNACK ____ A.M./P.M.			
Hunger:			
Fullness:			
	MEAL TOTALS		
DINNER ____ A.M./P.M.			
Hunger:			
Fullness:			
	MEAL TOTALS		
	DAILY TOTALS		

EXERCISE NOTES
_____ minutes

DAILY WRAP-UP
Goals: Exceeded ____ Met ____ Keep Trying ____
Notes:

Success Of The Day:

RESEARCH REPORT: When participants in a study ate a first course of low-calorie soup before a lunch entrée, they reduced their total calorie intake at lunch (soup and entrée) by 20 percent, compared to when they did not eat soup.

TUESDAY

SUPPLEMENTS [ ] [ ] WEIGHT [ ]

Today's Goals:

MEAL	FOODS & BEVERAGES	FOCUS I:	FOCUS 2:
BREAKFAST ___ A.M./P.M.			
Hunger:			
Fullness:			
	MEAL TOTALS		
SNACK ___ A.M./P.M.			
Hunger:			
Fullness:			
	MEAL TOTALS		
LUNCH ___ A.M./P.M.			
Hunger:			
Fullness:			
	MEAL TOTALS		
SNACK ___ A.M./P.M.			
Hunger:			
Fullness:			
	MEAL TOTALS		
DINNER ___ A.M./P.M.			
Hunger:			
Fullness:			
	MEAL TOTALS		
	DAILY TOTALS		

EXERCISE NOTES
_____ minutes

DAILY WRAP-UP
Goals: Exceeded ___ Met ___ Keep Trying ___
Notes:

Success Of The Day:

FOOD FACTOID: Eating together as a family on a regular basis lowers a child's obesity rate, promotes family bonding, and lets you model healthy eating habits.

FRIDAY

SUPPLEMENTS ☐ ☐   WEIGHT ☐

Today's Goals: _____

MEAL	FOODS & BEVERAGES	FOCUS I:	FOCUS 2:
BREAKFAST ____ A.M./P.M.			
Hunger:			
Fullness:			
	MEAL TOTALS		
SNACK ____ A.M./P.M.			
Hunger:			
Fullness:			
	MEAL TOTALS		
LUNCH ____ A.M./P.M.			
Hunger:			
Fullness:			
	MEAL TOTALS		
SNACK ____ A.M./P.M.			
Hunger:			
Fullness:			
	MEAL TOTALS		
DINNER ____ A.M./P.M.			
Hunger:			
Fullness:			
	MEAL TOTALS		
	DAILY TOTALS		

EXERCISE NOTES
_____ minutes

DAILY WRAP-UP
Goals: Exceeded ____ Met ____ Keep Trying ____

Notes:

Success Of The Day:

NUTRITION TIP: Be careful how you order sushi. So-called new wave sushis, including tempuras and rolls made with creamy sauces, fatty meats, and cheeses, can provide 500 or more calories per roll. Sushis made with steamed rice, fish, and vegetables contain 100 to 200 calories per roll.

SATURDAY

SUPPLEMENTS ☐ ☐   WEIGHT ☐

Today's Goals: _____

MEAL	FOODS & BEVERAGES		FOCUS 1:	FOCUS 2:
BREAKFAST ___ A.M./P.M.				
Hunger:				
Fullness:	MEAL TOTALS			
SNACK ___ A.M./P.M.				
Hunger:				
Fullness:	MEAL TOTALS			
LUNCH ___ A.M./P.M.				
Hunger:				
Fullness:	MEAL TOTALS			
SNACK ___ A.M./P.M.				
Hunger:				
Fullness:	MEAL TOTALS			
DINNER ___ A.M./P.M.				
Hunger:				
Fullness:	MEAL TOTALS			
	DAILY TOTALS			

EXERCISE NOTES
_____ minutes

DAILY WRAP-UP
Goals: Exceeded ___ Met ___ Keep Trying ___
Notes:

Success Of The Day:

FITNESS FACTOID: Amish men, who have a 0 percent obesity rate, walk more than 18,000 steps a day, and Amish women, with a 9 percent obesity rate, average more than 14,000 steps. Adults in Colorado, one of the leanest states, report taking 6,800 steps per day.

SUNDAY

SUPPLEMENTS ☐ ☐   WEIGHT ☐

Today's Goals: _____

MEAL	FOODS & BEVERAGES	FOCUS 1:	FOCUS 2:
BREAKFAST ___ A.M./P.M.			
Hunger:			
Fullness:			
	MEAL TOTALS		
SNACK ___ A.M./P.M.			
Hunger:			
Fullness:			
	MEAL TOTALS		
LUNCH ___ A.M./P.M.			
Hunger:			
Fullness:			
	MEAL TOTALS		
SNACK ___ A.M./P.M.			
Hunger:			
Fullness:			
	MEAL TOTALS		
DINNER ___ A.M./P.M.			
Hunger:			
Fullness:			
	MEAL TOTALS		
	DAILY TOTALS		

EXERCISE NOTES
_____ minutes

DAILY WRAP-UP
Goals: Exceeded ___ Met ___ Keep Trying ___
Notes:

Success Of The Day:

"Husband to his wife: You could lose a lot of weight if you'd just carry all your diet books around the block once a day." — BILL HOEST, cartoonist

WEEKLY WRAP-UP

SUCCESS OF THE WEEK

GOALS ASSESSMENT

EXERCISE NOTES **TOTAL DAYS EXERCISED** [ ]   **TOTAL MINUTES/ HOURS** [ ]

PROGRESS REPORT

WHAT WENT WELL, AND WHY?

WHAT DIDN'T GO WELL? WHAT GOT IN MY WAY?

WHAT IS THE MOST IMPORTANT INSIGHT I GAINED ABOUT MYSELF THIS WEEK?

WHAT DO I PLAN TO DO DIFFERENTLY NEXT WEEK?

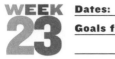

WEEK 23

Dates: _____

Goals for the Week: _____

_____

MONDAY

SUPPLEMENTS [ ] [ ]　WEIGHT [ ]

Today's Goals: _____

MEAL	FOODS & BEVERAGES	FOCUS 1:	FOCUS 2:
BREAKFAST ___ A.M./P.M.			
Hunger:			
Fullness:			
	MEAL TOTALS		
SNACK ___ A.M./P.M.			
Hunger:			
Fullness:			
	MEAL TOTALS		
LUNCH ___ A.M./P.M.			
Hunger:			
Fullness:			
	MEAL TOTALS		
SNACK ___ A.M./P.M.			
Hunger:			
Fullness:			
	MEAL TOTALS		
DINNER ___ A.M./P.M.			
Hunger:			
Fullness:			
	MEAL TOTALS		
	DAILY TOTALS		

EXERCISE NOTES
_____ minutes

DAILY WRAP-UP
Goals: Exceeded ___ Met ___ Keep Trying ___
Notes:

Success Of The Day:

RESEARCH REPORT: Breast cancer survivors who eat at least five servings of vegetables and fruits a day <u>and</u> walk briskly for 30 minutes, 6 days a week can reduce their risk of dying from breast cancer by half. This applies even to overweight women.

TUESDAY

SUPPLEMENTS ☐ ☐ WEIGHT ☐

Today's Goals: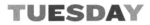

MEAL	FOODS & BEVERAGES	FOCUS I:	FOCUS 2:
BREAKFAST ___ A.M./P.M.			
Hunger:			
Fullness:	MEAL TOTALS		
SNACK ___ A.M./P.M.			
Hunger:			
Fullness:	MEAL TOTALS		
LUNCH ___ A.M./P.M.			
Hunger:			
Fullness:	MEAL TOTALS		
SNACK ___ A.M./P.M.			
Hunger:			
Fullness:	MEAL TOTALS		
DINNER ___ A.M./P.M.			
Hunger:			
Fullness:	MEAL TOTALS		
	DAILY TOTALS		

EXERCISE NOTES
_____ minutes

DAILY WRAP-UP
Goals: Exceeded ___ Met ___ Keep Trying ___
Notes:

Success Of The Day:

NUTRITION SHOCKER: On a typical diet, the maximum number of combined saturated and trans fat grams recommended per day is 22. A Burger King Whopper with cheese alone has 29 grams of artery-clogging fat.

WEDNESDAY   SUPPLEMENTS ☐ ☐   WEIGHT ☐

Today's Goals:

MEAL	FOODS & BEVERAGES	FOCUS I:	FOCUS 2:
BREAKFAST ___ A.M./P.M.			
Hunger:			
Fullness:			
	MEAL TOTALS		
SNACK ___ A.M./P.M.			
Hunger:			
Fullness:			
	MEAL TOTALS		
LUNCH ___ A.M./P.M.			
Hunger:			
Fullness:			
	MEAL TOTALS		
SNACK ___ A.M./P.M.			
Hunger:			
Fullness:			
	MEAL TOTALS		
DINNER ___ A.M./P.M.			
Hunger:			
Fullness:			
	MEAL TOTALS		
	DAILY TOTALS		

EXERCISE NOTES
_____ minutes

DAILY WRAP-UP
Goals: Exceeded ___ Met ___ Keep Trying ___
Notes:

Success Of The Day:

BY THE NUMBERS: 300. Percent of the Daily Value for vitamin C in one medium papaya. **140:** Calories in the papaya. **5.5:** Fiber grams. **100:** Percent of vitamin C in 11.5-ounce can of Kern's Nectar papaya juice. **210:** Calories in the juice. **0:** Fiber grams in the juice.

THURSDAY

SUPPLEMENTS ☐ ☐ WEIGHT ☐

Today's Goals:

MEAL	FOODS & BEVERAGES	FOCUS 1:	FOCUS 2:
BREAKFAST ___ A.M./P.M.			
Hunger:			
Fullness:			
	MEAL TOTALS		
SNACK ___ A.M./P.M.			
Hunger:			
Fullness:			
	MEAL TOTALS		
LUNCH ___ A.M./P.M.			
Hunger:			
Fullness:			
	MEAL TOTALS		
SNACK ___ A.M./P.M.			
Hunger:			
Fullness:			
	MEAL TOTALS		
DINNER ___ A.M./P.M.			
Hunger:			
Fullness:			
	MEAL TOTALS		
	DAILY TOTALS		

EXERCISE NOTES
_____ minutes

DAILY WRAP-UP
Goals: Exceeded ___ Met ___ Keep Trying ___
Notes:

Success Of The Day:

FOOD FACTOID: We taste before we're born. Food chemicals with distinct tastes and smells are transmitted to the amniotic fluid that cushions a growing baby. The fetus swallows this fluid and can sense the flavors.

FRIDAY

SUPPLEMENTS ☐ ☐   WEIGHT ☐

Today's Goals:

MEAL	FOODS & BEVERAGES	FOCUS I:	FOCUS 2:
BREAKFAST ___ A.M./P.M.			
Hunger:			
Fullness:			
	MEAL TOTALS		
SNACK ___ A.M./P.M.			
Hunger:			
Fullness:			
	MEAL TOTALS		
LUNCH ___ A.M./P.M.			
Hunger:			
Fullness:			
	MEAL TOTALS		
SNACK ___ A.M./P.M.			
Hunger:			
Fullness:			
	MEAL TOTALS		
DINNER ___ A.M./P.M.			
Hunger:			
Fullness:			
	MEAL TOTALS		
	DAILY TOTALS		

EXERCISE NOTES
_____ minutes

DAILY WRAP-UP
Goals: Exceeded ___ Met ___ Keep Trying ___
Notes:

Success Of The Day:

NUTRITION TIP: Just 2 percent of the wheat flour Americans eat is consumed as whole wheat. When you shop this week, swap out one refined grain product — hamburger buns, bagels, pitas, flour tortillas, pasta, or crackers — for a whole-wheat version.

SATURDAY

SUPPLEMENTS ☐ ☐   WEIGHT ☐

Today's Goals:

MEAL	FOODS & BEVERAGES	FOCUS 1:	FOCUS 2:
BREAKFAST ____ A.M./P.M.			
Hunger:			
Fullness:			
	MEAL TOTALS		
SNACK ____ A.M./P.M.			
Hunger:			
Fullness:			
	MEAL TOTALS		
LUNCH ____ A.M./P.M.			
Hunger:			
Fullness:			
	MEAL TOTALS		
SNACK ____ A.M./P.M.			
Hunger:			
Fullness:			
	MEAL TOTALS		
DINNER ____ A.M./P.M.			
Hunger:			
Fullness:			
	MEAL TOTALS		
	DAILY TOTALS		

EXERCISE NOTES
_____ minutes

DAILY WRAP-UP
Goals: Exceeded ___   Met ___   Keep Trying ___
Notes:

Success Of The Day:

FITNESS FACTOID: Lifting weights improves balance. In a 1-year study, middle-aged women who didn't exercise showed an 8.5 percent decline in balance, whereas those who lifted weights improved their balance by 14 percent.

SUNDAY

SUPPLEMENTS ☐ ☐   WEIGHT ☐

Today's Goals:

MEAL	FOODS & BEVERAGES	FOCUS I:	FOCUS 2:
BREAKFAST ___ A.M./P.M.			
Hunger:			
Fullness:	MEAL TOTALS		
SNACK ___ A.M./P.M.			
Hunger:			
Fullness:	MEAL TOTALS		
LUNCH ___ A.M./P.M.			
Hunger:			
Fullness:	MEAL TOTALS		
SNACK ___ A.M./P.M.			
Hunger:			
Fullness:	MEAL TOTALS		
DINNER ___ A.M./P.M.			
Hunger:			
Fullness:	MEAL TOTALS		
	DAILY TOTALS		

EXERCISE NOTES
_____ minutes

DAILY WRAP-UP
Goals: Exceeded ___ Met ___ Keep Trying ___
Notes:

Success Of The Day:

"We're the country that has more food to eat than any other country in the world, and with more diets to keep us from eating it." — AUTHOR UNKNOWN

WEEKLY WRAP-UP

SUCCESS OF THE WEEK

GOALS ASSESSMENT

EXERCISE NOTES　　　　**TOTAL DAYS EXERCISED** [　　]　　**TOTAL MINUTES/ HOURS** [　　]

PROGRESS REPORT

WHAT WENT WELL, AND WHY?

WHAT DIDN'T GO WELL? WHAT GOT IN MY WAY?

WHAT IS THE MOST IMPORTANT INSIGHT I GAINED ABOUT MYSELF THIS WEEK?

WHAT DO I PLAN TO DO DIFFERENTLY NEXT WEEK?

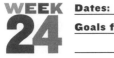

WEEK 24

Dates: _____

Goals for the Week: _____

_____

MONDAY

SUPPLEMENTS ☐☐   WEIGHT ☐

Today's Goals: _____

MEAL	FOODS & BEVERAGES	FOCUS I:	FOCUS 2:
BREAKFAST ___ A.M./P.M.			
Hunger:			
Fullness:	MEAL TOTALS		
SNACK ___ A.M./P.M.			
Hunger:			
Fullness:	MEAL TOTALS		
LUNCH ___ A.M./P.M.			
Hunger:			
Fullness:	MEAL TOTALS		
SNACK ___ A.M./P.M.			
Hunger:			
Fullness:	MEAL TOTALS		
DINNER ___ A.M./P.M.			
Hunger:			
Fullness:	MEAL TOTALS		
	DAILY TOTALS		

EXERCISE NOTES
_____ minutes

DAILY WRAP-UP
Goals: Exceeded ___ Met ___ Keep Trying ___
Notes:
Success Of The Day:

RESEARCH REPORT: The more foods and flavors we're exposed to — think Las Vegas buffets — the more we eat. In several studies, subjects ate significantly more yogurt, sandwiches, and ice cream when offered several flavors than when offered a single flavor.

TUESDAY

SUPPLEMENTS ☐ ☐   WEIGHT ☐

Today's Goals:

MEAL	FOODS & BEVERAGES	FOCUS I:	FOCUS 2:
BREAKFAST ___ A.M./P.M.			
Hunger:			
Fullness:	MEAL TOTALS		
SNACK ___ A.M./P.M.			
Hunger:			
Fullness:	MEAL TOTALS		
LUNCH ___ A.M./P.M.			
Hunger:			
Fullness:	MEAL TOTALS		
SNACK ___ A.M./P.M.			
Hunger:			
Fullness:	MEAL TOTALS		
DINNER ___ A.M./P.M.			
Hunger:			
Fullness:	MEAL TOTALS		
	DAILY TOTALS		

EXERCISE NOTES
_____ minutes

DAILY WRAP-UP
Goals: Exceeded ___ Met ___ Keep Trying ___
Notes:

Success Of The Day:

NUTRITION SHOCKER: In the 1950s, a typical fast-food restaurant served an 8-ounce soft drink. Today the "child size" is 12 ounces, while large sizes range from 30 to 40 ounces.

WEDNESDAY

SUPPLEMENTS ☐ ☐   WEIGHT ☐

Today's Goals:

MEAL	FOODS & BEVERAGES	FOCUS I:	FOCUS 2:
BREAKFAST ____ A.M./P.M.			
Hunger:			
Fullness:	MEAL TOTALS		
SNACK ____ A.M./P.M.			
Hunger:			
Fullness:	MEAL TOTALS		
LUNCH ____ A.M./P.M.			
Hunger:			
Fullness:	MEAL TOTALS		
SNACK ____ A.M./P.M.			
Hunger:			
Fullness:	MEAL TOTALS		
DINNER ____ A.M./P.M.			
Hunger:			
Fullness:	MEAL TOTALS		
	DAILY TOTALS		

EXERCISE NOTES
_____ minutes

DAILY WRAP-UP
Goals: Exceeded ____ Met ____ Keep Trying ____
Notes:

Success Of The Day:

BY THE NUMBERS: 425: Weight, in pounds, of Jared Fogle before he started eating all meals at Subway. **190:** Jared's weight one year later. **280:** Calories in Jared's daily lunch, a turkey sub (no mayo or cheese), with Baked Lay's. **450:** Calories in Jared's daily dinner, the foot-long veggie sub.

THURSDAY

SUPPLEMENTS ☐ ☐   WEIGHT ☐

Today's Goals:

MEAL	FOODS & BEVERAGES	FOCUS I:	FOCUS 2:
BREAKFAST ___ A.M./P.M.			
Hunger:			
Fullness:	MEAL TOTALS		
SNACK ___ A.M./P.M.			
Hunger:			
Fullness:	MEAL TOTALS		
LUNCH ___ A.M./P.M.			
Hunger:			
Fullness:	MEAL TOTALS		
SNACK ___ A.M./P.M			
Hunger:			
Fullness:	MEAL TOTALS		
DINNER ___ A.M./P.M.			
Hunger:			
Fullness:	MEAL TOTALS		
	DAILY TOTALS		

EXERCISE NOTES
_____ minutes

DAILY WRAP-UP
Goals: Exceeded ___ Met ___ Keep Trying ___
Notes:

Success Of The Day:

FOOD FACTOID: The top-selling condiment in the United States isn't ketchup. According to the Association for Dressings and Sauces, salsa displaced ketchup as number I in the year 2000.

FRIDAY

SUPPLEMENTS ☐ ☐   WEIGHT ☐

Today's Goals:

MEAL	FOODS & BEVERAGES	FOCUS 1:	FOCUS 2:
BREAKFAST ___ A.M./P.M.			
Hunger:			
Fullness:			
	MEAL TOTALS		
SNACK ___ A.M./P.M.			
Hunger:			
Fullness:			
	MEAL TOTALS		
LUNCH ___ A.M./P.M.			
Hunger:			
Fullness:			
	MEAL TOTALS		
SNACK ___ A.M./P.M.			
Hunger:			
Fullness:			
	MEAL TOTALS		
DINNER ___ A.M./P.M.			
Hunger:			
Fullness:			
	MEAL TOTALS		
	DAILY TOTALS		

EXERCISE NOTES
_____ minutes

DAILY WRAP-UP
Goals: Exceeded ___ Met ___ Keep Trying ___
Notes:

Success Of The Day:

NUTRITION TIP: Cheese is America's top source of saturated fat, and consumption has tripled since 1970. Try replacing whole-milk cheese with reduced-fat versions of Swiss, feta, mozzarella, cottage, and ricotta.

SATURDAY

SUPPLEMENTS ☐ ☐ WEIGHT ☐

Today's Goals:

MEAL	FOODS & BEVERAGES		FOCUS 1:	FOCUS 2:
BREAKFAST ___ A.M./P.M.				
Hunger:				
Fullness:		MEAL TOTALS		
SNACK ___ A.M./P.M.				
Hunger:				
Fullness:		MEAL TOTALS		
LUNCH ___ A.M./P.M.				
Hunger:				
Fullness:		MEAL TOTALS		
SNACK ___ A.M./P.M.				
Hunger:				
Fullness:		MEAL TOTALS		
DINNER ___ A.M./P.M.				
Hunger:				
Fullness:		MEAL TOTALS		
		DAILY TOTALS		

EXERCISE NOTES
_____ minutes

DAILY WRAP-UP
Goals: Exceeded ___ Met ___ Keep Trying ___
Notes:

Success Of The Day:

FITNESS FACTOID: Pumping iron may be as good for your heart as it is for your muscles. In one study, men who lifted weights at least 30 minutes a week had a 23 percent lower heart-disease risk than men who didn't lift.

SUNDAY

SUPPLEMENTS ☐ ☐   WEIGHT ☐

Today's Goals:

MEAL	FOODS & BEVERAGES	FOCUS I:	FOCUS 2:
BREAKFAST ____ A.M./P.M.			
Hunger:			
Fullness:			
	MEAL TOTALS		
SNACK ____ A.M./P.M.			
Hunger:			
Fullness:			
	MEAL TOTALS		
LUNCH ____ A.M./P.M.			
Hunger:			
Fullness:			
	MEAL TOTALS		
SNACK ____ A.M./P.M.			
Hunger:			
Fullness:			
	MEAL TOTALS		
DINNER ____ A.M./P.M.			
Hunger:			
Fullness:			
	MEAL TOTALS		
	DAILY TOTALS		

EXERCISE NOTES
_____ minutes

DAILY WRAP-UP
Goals: Exceeded ____ Met ____ Keep Trying ____
Notes:

Success Of The Day:

"If you have formed the habit of checking on every new diet that comes along, you will find that, mercifully, they all blur together, leaving you with only one definite piece of information: french-fried potatoes are out."

— JEAN KERR, author

WEEKLY WRAP-UP

SUCCESS OF THE WEEK

GOALS ASSESSMENT

EXERCISE NOTES   **TOTAL DAYS EXERCISED**   **TOTAL MINUTES/ HOURS**

PROGRESS REPORT

WHAT WENT WELL, AND WHY?

WHAT DIDN'T GO WELL? WHAT GOT IN MY WAY?

WHAT IS THE MOST IMPORTANT INSIGHT I GAINED ABOUT MYSELF THIS WEEK?

WHAT DO I PLAN TO DO DIFFERENTLY NEXT WEEK?

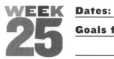

WEEK 25

Dates: _____

Goals for the Week: _____

_____

MONDAY

SUPPLEMENTS ☐ ☐   WEIGHT ☐

Today's Goals: _____

MEAL	FOODS & BEVERAGES	FOCUS 1:	FOCUS 2:
BREAKFAST ___ A.M./P.M.			
Hunger:			
Fullness:			
	MEAL TOTALS		
SNACK ___ A.M./P.M.			
Hunger:			
Fullness:			
	MEAL TOTALS		
LUNCH ___ A.M./P.M.			
Hunger:			
Fullness:			
	MEAL TOTALS		
SNACK ___ A.M./P.M.			
Hunger:			
Fullness:			
	MEAL TOTALS		
DINNER ___ A.M./P.M.			
Hunger:			
Fullness:			
	MEAL TOTALS		
	DAILY TOTALS		

EXERCISE NOTES
_____ minutes

DAILY WRAP-UP
Goals: Exceeded ___ Met ___ Keep Trying ___
Notes:

Success Of The Day:

RESEARCH REPORT: The more kids watch TV, the more calories they eat — 167 calories for each extra hour viewed, according to one study. One-third of all 6- and 7-year-old children in the United States have a TV in their bedroom.

TUESDAY

SUPPLEMENTS ☐ ☐   WEIGHT ☐

Today's Goals:

MEAL	FOODS & BEVERAGES	FOCUS 1:	FOCUS 2:
BREAKFAST ___ A.M./P.M.			
Hunger:			
Fullness:			
	MEAL TOTALS		
SNACK ___ A.M./P.M.			
Hunger:			
Fullness:			
	MEAL TOTALS		
LUNCH ___ A.M./P.M.			
Hunger:			
Fullness:			
	MEAL TOTALS		
SNACK ___ A.M./P.M.			
Hunger:			
Fullness:			
	MEAL TOTALS		
DINNER ___ A.M./P.M.			
Hunger:			
Fullness:			
	MEAL TOTALS		
	DAILY TOTALS		

EXERCISE NOTES
_____ minutes

DAILY WRAP-UP
Goals: Exceeded ___   Met ___   Keep Trying ___
Notes:

Success Of The Day:

NUTRITION SHOCKER: Twenty-five years ago, teenagers drank almost twice as much milk as soda pop. Today they drink twice as much soda as milk.

WEDNESDAY   SUPPLEMENTS ☐ ☐   WEIGHT ☐

Today's Goals:

MEAL	FOODS & BEVERAGES	FOCUS I:	FOCUS 2:
BREAKFAST ___ A.M./P.M.			
Hunger:			
Fullness:			
	MEAL TOTALS		
SNACK ___ A.M./P.M.			
Hunger:			
Fullness:			
	MEAL TOTALS		
LUNCH ___ A.M./P.M.			
Hunger:			
Fullness:			
	MEAL TOTALS		
SNACK ___ A.M./P.M.			
Hunger:			
Fullness:			
	MEAL TOTALS		
DINNER ___ A.M./P.M.			
Hunger:			
Fullness:			
	MEAL TOTALS		
	DAILY TOTALS		

EXERCISE NOTES
_____ minutes

DAILY WRAP-UP
Goals: Exceeded ___ Met ___ Keep Trying ___
Notes:

Success Of The Day:

BY THE NUMBERS: **2,400:** Years since Hippocrates wrote, "Everything in excess is opposed to nature." **4:** Years since a government official said today's kids are the first generation who will have a shorter life span than their parents if we don't change our lifestyle.

THURSDAY

SUPPLEMENTS ☐☐ WEIGHT ☐

Today's Goals:

MEAL	FOODS & BEVERAGES	FOCUS 1:	FOCUS 2:
BREAKFAST __ A.M./P.M.			
Hunger:			
Fullness:	MEAL TOTALS		
SNACK __ A.M./P.M.			
Hunger:			
Fullness:	MEAL TOTALS		
LUNCH __ A.M./P.M.			
Hunger:			
Fullness:	MEAL TOTALS		
SNACK __ A.M./P.M.			
Hunger:			
Fullness:	MEAL TOTALS		
DINNER __ A.M./P.M.			
Hunger:			
Fullness:	MEAL TOTALS		
	DAILY TOTALS		

EXERCISE NOTES
_____ minutes

DAILY WRAP-UP
Goals: Exceeded ___ Met ___ Keep Trying ___
Notes:

Success Of The Day:

FOOD FACTOID: Adolescents who play sports have better eating habits than inactive youth, eating breakfast more frequently and consuming more protein, calcium, and iron.

FRIDAY

SUPPLEMENTS ☐ ☐   WEIGHT ☐

Today's Goals:

MEAL	FOODS & BEVERAGES	FOCUS I:	FOCUS 2:
BREAKFAST ___ A.M./P.M.			
Hunger:			
Fullness:			
	MEAL TOTALS		
SNACK ___ A.M./P.M.			
Hunger:			
Fullness:			
	MEAL TOTALS		
LUNCH ___ A.M./P.M.			
Hunger:			
Fullness:			
	MEAL TOTALS		
SNACK ___ A.M./P.M.			
Hunger:			
Fullness:			
	MEAL TOTALS		
DINNER ___ A.M./P.M.			
Hunger:			
Fullness:			
	MEAL TOTALS		
	DAILY TOTALS		

EXERCISE NOTES
_____ minutes

DAILY WRAP-UP
Goals: Exceeded ___ Met ___ Keep Trying ___
Notes:

Success Of The Day:

NUTRITION TIP: Since smaller plates and utensils lead to eating smaller portions, try downsizing your dining set by scouting garage sales for an old-fashioned petite place setting. Or have some fun and buy a kids' set with your favorite character.

SATURDAY

SUPPLEMENTS ☐ ☐   WEIGHT ☐

Today's Goals:

MEAL	FOODS & BEVERAGES	FOCUS I:	FOCUS 2:
BREAKFAST ___ A.M./P.M.			
Hunger:			
Fullness:			
	MEAL TOTALS		
SNACK ___ A.M./P.M.			
Hunger:			
Fullness:			
	MEAL TOTALS		
LUNCH ___ A.M./P.M.			
Hunger:			
Fullness:			
	MEAL TOTALS		
SNACK ___ A.M./P.M.			
Hunger:			
Fullness:			
	MEAL TOTALS		
DINNER ___ A.M./P.M.			
Hunger:			
Fullness:			
	MEAL TOTALS		
	DAILY TOTALS		

EXERCISE NOTES
_____ minutes

DAILY WRAP-UP
Goals: Exceeded ___ Met ___ Keep Trying ___
Notes:

Success Of The Day:

FITNESS FACTOID: Physically active men and women may be **40** to **50** percent less likely to develop colon cancer than couch potatoes. Active women may be **30** to **40** percent less likely to develop breast cancer. It's also likely that exercise reduces the risk of lung, endometrial, and prostate cancers.

SUNDAY

SUPPLEMENTS ☐ ☐   WEIGHT ☐

Today's Goals:

MEAL	FOODS & BEVERAGES	FOCUS 1:	FOCUS 2:
BREAKFAST ____ A.M./P.M.			
Hunger:			
Fullness:			
	MEAL TOTALS		
SNACK ____ A.M./P.M.			
Hunger:			
Fullness:			
	MEAL TOTALS		
LUNCH ____ A.M./P.M.			
Hunger:			
Fullness:			
	MEAL TOTALS		
SNACK ____ A.M./P.M.			
Hunger:			
Fullness:			
	MEAL TOTALS		
DINNER ____ A.M./P.M.			
Hunger:			
Fullness:			
	MEAL TOTALS		
	DAILY TOTALS		

EXERCISE NOTES
_____ minutes

DAILY WRAP-UP
Goals: Exceeded ____ Met ____ Keep Trying ____
Notes:

Success Of The Day:

"Another good reducing exercise consists of placing both hands against the table edge and pushing back."
— ROBERT QUILLEN

WEEKLY WRAP-UP

SUCCESS OF THE WEEK

GOALS ASSESSMENT

EXERCISE NOTES   TOTAL DAYS EXERCISED [   ]   TOTAL MINUTES/ HOURS [   ]

PROGRESS REPORT

WHAT WENT WELL, AND WHY?

WHAT DIDN'T GO WELL? WHAT GOT IN MY WAY?

WHAT IS THE MOST IMPORTANT INSIGHT I GAINED ABOUT MYSELF THIS WEEK?

WHAT DO I PLAN TO DO DIFFERENTLY NEXT WEEK?

WEEK
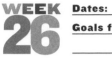 **26**

Dates: _____

Goals for the Week: _____

_____

MONDAY

SUPPLEMENTS ☐ ☐ WEIGHT ☐

Today's Goals: _____

MEAL	FOODS & BEVERAGES	FOCUS I:	FOCUS 2:
BREAKFAST ____ A.M./P.M.			
Hunger:			
Fullness:			
	MEAL TOTALS		
SNACK ____ A.M./P.M.			
Hunger:			
Fullness:			
	MEAL TOTALS		
LUNCH ____ A.M./P.M.			
Hunger:			
Fullness:			
	MEAL TOTALS		
SNACK ____ A.M./P.M.			
Hunger:			
Fullness:			
	MEAL TOTALS		
DINNER ____ A.M./P.M.			
Hunger:			
Fullness:			
	MEAL TOTALS		
	DAILY TOTALS		

EXERCISE NOTES
_____ minutes

DAILY WRAP-UP
Goals: Exceeded ____ Met ____ Keep Trying ____
Notes:

Success Of The Day:

RESEARCH REPORT: Eating consistently aids weight management. People who consume roughly the same number of calories daily are 150 percent more likely to maintain their weight than those who vary their calorie intake each day.

TUESDAY

SUPPLEMENTS ☐ ☐   WEIGHT ☐

Today's Goals:

MEAL	FOODS & BEVERAGES	FOCUS 1:	FOCUS 2:
BREAKFAST ___ A.M./P.M.			
Hunger:			
Fullness:			
	MEAL TOTALS		
SNACK ___ A.M./P.M.			
Hunger:			
Fullness:			
	MEAL TOTALS		
LUNCH ___ A.M./P.M.			
Hunger:			
Fullness:			
	MEAL TOTALS		
SNACK ___ A.M./P.M.			
Hunger:			
Fullness:			
	MEAL TOTALS		
DINNER ___ A.M./P.M.			
Hunger:			
Fullness:			
	MEAL TOTALS		
	DAILY TOTALS		

EXERCISE NOTES
_____ minutes

DAILY WRAP-UP
Goals: Exceeded ___ Met ___ Keep Trying ___
Notes:

Success Of The Day:

NUTRITION SHOCKER: In China, the most recognized non-Chinese corporate symbol is the KFC logo. The prevalence of obesity in China has doubled in the last 10 years.

WEDNESDAY SUPPLEMENTS ☐ ☐ WEIGHT ☐

Today's Goals:

MEAL	FOODS & BEVERAGES	FOCUS 1:	FOCUS 2:
BREAKFAST ____ A.M./P.M.			
Hunger:			
Fullness:	MEAL TOTALS		
SNACK ____ A.M./P.M.			
Hunger:			
Fullness:	MEAL TOTALS		
LUNCH ____ A.M./P.M.			
Hunger:			
Fullness:	MEAL TOTALS		
SNACK ____ A.M./P.M.			
Hunger:			
Fullness:	MEAL TOTALS		
DINNER ____ A.M./P.M.			
Hunger:			
Fullness:	MEAL TOTALS		
	DAILY TOTALS		

EXERCISE NOTES
_____ minutes

DAILY WRAP-UP
Goals: Exceeded ____ Met ____ Keep Trying ____
Notes:

Success Of The Day:

BY THE NUMBERS: **160°F:** Temperature red meat must be cooked to in order to kill bacteria. **170°F:** Temperature for chicken. **2:** Maximum hours perishable food can be left at room temperature.

THURSDAY

SUPPLEMENTS ☐ ☐ WEIGHT ☐

Today's Goals:

MEAL	FOODS & BEVERAGES	FOCUS 1:	FOCUS 2:
BREAKFAST			
____ A.M./P.M.			
Hunger:			
Fullness:			
	MEAL TOTALS		
SNACK			
____ A.M./P.M.			
Hunger:			
Fullness:			
	MEAL TOTALS		
LUNCH			
____ A.M./P.M.			
Hunger:			
Fullness:			
	MEAL TOTALS		
SNACK			
____ A.M./P.M.			
Hunger:			
Fullness:			
	MEAL TOTALS		
DINNER			
____ A.M./P.M.			
Hunger:			
Fullness:			
	MEAL TOTALS		
	DAILY TOTALS		

EXERCISE NOTES
_____ minutes

DAILY WRAP-UP
Goals: Exceeded ____ Met ____ Keep Trying ____
Notes:

Success Of The Day:

FOOD FACTOID: Women who get most of their daily calcium from food have healthier bones than women whose calcium comes mainly from supplements. Calcium from the diet is generally better absorbed than supplementary calcium.

FRIDAY

SUPPLEMENTS ☐ ☐   WEIGHT ☐

Today's Goals:

MEAL	FOODS & BEVERAGES	FOCUS I:	FOCUS 2:
BREAKFAST ____ A.M./P.M.			
Hunger:			
Fullness:	MEAL TOTALS		
SNACK ____ A.M./P.M.			
Hunger:			
Fullness:	MEAL TOTALS		
LUNCH ____ A.M./P.M.			
Hunger:			
Fullness:	MEAL TOTALS		
SNACK ____ A.M./P.M.			
Hunger:			
Fullness:	MEAL TOTALS		
DINNER ____ A.M./P.M.			
Hunger:			
Fullness:	MEAL TOTALS		
	DAILY TOTALS		

EXERCISE NOTES
_____ minutes

DAILY WRAP-UP
Goals: Exceeded ____ Met ____ Keep Trying ____
Notes:

Success Of The Day:

NUTRITION TIP: Though our bodies can make vitamin D through sun exposure, a recent study found that 5 percent of Hawaiians who spend 20 to 30 hours per week outdoors had low vitamin D levels. Look for vitamin D–fortified foods such as orange juice or cereal.

SATURDAY

SUPPLEMENTS ☐ ☐   WEIGHT ☐

Today's Goals:

MEAL	FOODS & BEVERAGES	FOCUS I:	FOCUS 2:
BREAKFAST ____ A.M./P.M.			
Hunger:			
Fullness:			
	MEAL TOTALS		
SNACK ____ A.M./P.M.			
Hunger:			
Fullness:			
	MEAL TOTALS		
LUNCH ____ A.M./P.M.			
Hunger:			
Fullness:			
	MEAL TOTALS		
SNACK ____ A.M./P.M.			
Hunger:			
Fullness:			
	MEAL TOTALS		
DINNER ____ A.M./P.M.			
Hunger:			
Fullness:			
	MEAL TOTALS		
	DAILY TOTALS		

EXERCISE NOTES
_____ minutes

DAILY WRAP-UP
Goals: Exceeded ____   Met ____   Keep Trying ____
Notes:

Success Of The Day:

FITNESS FACTOID: It's not true that long, slow workouts are better for weight loss than shorter, more intense ones. What matters is how many calories you burn. The best strategy for weight loss, fitness, and injury prevention is to vary your pace and distance.

SUNDAY

SUPPLEMENTS ☐ ☐ WEIGHT ☐

Today's Goals: _____

MEAL	FOODS & BEVERAGES	FOCUS I:	FOCUS 2:
BREAKFAST ____ A.M./P.M.			
Hunger:			
Fullness:			
	MEAL TOTALS		
SNACK ____ A.M./P.M.			
Hunger:			
Fullness:			
	MEAL TOTALS		
LUNCH ____ A.M./P.M.			
Hunger:			
Fullness:			
	MEAL TOTALS		
SNACK ____ A.M./P.M.			
Hunger:			
Fullness:			
	MEAL TOTALS		
DINNER ____ A.M./P.M.			
Hunger:			
Fullness:			
	MEAL TOTALS		
	DAILY TOTALS		

EXERCISE NOTES
_____ minutes

DAILY WRAP-UP
Goals: Exceeded ____ Met ____ Keep Trying ____
Notes:

Success Of The Day:

"Stressed spelled backwards is desserts. Coincidence? I think not!"

—AUTHOR UNKNOWN

WEEKLY WRAP-UP

SUCCESS OF THE WEEK

GOALS ASSESSMENT

EXERCISE NOTES   **TOTAL DAYS EXERCISED**   **TOTAL MINUTES/ HOURS**

PROGRESS REPORT

WHAT WENT WELL, AND WHY?

WHAT DIDN'T GO WELL? WHAT GOT IN MY WAY?

WHAT IS THE MOST IMPORTANT INSIGHT I GAINED ABOUT MYSELF THIS WEEK?

WHAT DO I PLAN TO DO DIFFERENTLY NEXT WEEK?

Charting Your Weight

Use the following chart to document your weight loss over the twenty-six weeks of the log. In the vertical column on the left, fill in a range of weights starting three to five pounds heavier than you are now and dropping down to your twenty-six-week goal weight in half-pound increments.

No, we don't expect you to gain three to five pounds! But weight fluctuations are normal. When you step on the scale, you're weighing everything that has weight, not just muscle, bone, and body fat, but also water, undigested food (even if it will all be burned off later), and waste your body hasn't eliminated yet. Your weight can shift quickly, from day to day or hour to hour, even if your muscle and body fat remain exactly the same.

Though you may weigh yourself daily, choose one day of the week to fill in this chart. Look for a pattern over time instead of focusing on every spike and dip. If the pattern is moving in the wrong direction, take a hard look at your log and reevaluate your strategies.

WEEK	1	2	3	4	5	6	7	8	9	10	11	12
WEIGHT												

13	14	15	16	17	18	19	20	21	22	23	24	25	26